The *New* Total Rider

HEALTH & FITNESS FOR THE EQUESTRIAN

The *New* Total Rider

HEALTH & FITNESS FOR THE EQUESTRIAN

Tom Holmes

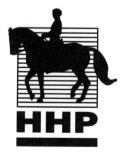

Half Halt Press, Inc.
Boonsboro, Maryland 21713

The New Total Rider:
Health & Fitness for the Equestrian

©2001 Tom Holmes

Published in the United States of America by
Half Halt Press, Inc.
P.O. Box 67
Boonsboro, MD 21713
www.halfhaltpress.com

Cover & text design by Olive Holmes
Cover illustration by Shan Wells
Text illustrations by Shan Wells, Susan Wood, Tom Holmes and Olive Holmes

ACKNOWLEDGMENTS

THE AUTHOR WOULD LIKE TO THANK the following people for their invaluable contributions to this book. Their knowledge, inspiration, commitment and generosity made this book and its success possible:

Jennifer Anderson, Ph.D., R.D. – nutrition extension specialist, Department of Food Science and Human Nutrition, Colorado State University

Karen Bannister – trainer and rider of multiple APHA National and World Champions

Barbara J. Beck, Ph.D. – health and fitness specialist, and equestrian

Katie Beck – Saddleseat Equitation Champion and U.S. Nationals Top-20 rider in Saddleseat Equitation and Ladies Sidesaddle

Elizabeth Carnes – publisher (Half Halt Press, Inc.) and friend

Cyndi Castiglioni – fitness instructor and illustration model

Dr. Deepak Chopra – world-renowned western and Ayurvedic physician and author

Marilyn Colter – consultant

Bob Culver – kinesiologist, personal trainer, illustration model and friend

Phyllis Dawson – USET member; highest placing American equestrian in 1988 Olympics in Seoul, Korea

Terri Fithian – fitness instructor and illustration model

Frank Fristensky – personal trainer

Caroline Gabriel – naturopathic nutritionist

Todd Gross – illustration model

Troy Heikes – trainer and rider of multiple APHA National and World Reining Champions, Freestyle Reining Champions, Jumping Champion, APHA Superhorse, and NHRA World Freestyle Reining Champion

Barb Hermsen – certified fitness and conditioning instructor

Olive Holmes – beloved wife, dearest friend, source of continuous inspiration and motivation, and book designer

Debbie Horzepa – illustration model

Ellene Busch-Kloepfer – dressage rider and instructor

Dr. Vasant Lad – world-renowned Ayurvedic physician and author

Pilar Gutierrez Martin – Ayurvedic practitioner, Creating Health Instructor and dear friend

Margot Nacey, Ed.D. – licensed clinical psychologist, equine sport psychologist and equestrian

Tanya Nuhsbaum – fitness instructor, illustration model and equestrian

Bill Robertson – USET member from 1962-1963 and renowned show jumping instructor

Kay Roth, Ph.D. – exercise physiologist

Shawn Scholl, M.S. – exercise physiologist, fitness instructor and competitive cyclist

Dr. Robert Svoboda – world-renowned Ayurvedic physician and author

Charles Throckmorton – trainer and rider of multiple Colorado Open Jumping Champions

Craig Vandegrift – certified fitness instructor and competitive bodybuilder

Steve Wade, M.S. – physical therapist

Mary Walhood – dressage rider and instructor

Shan Wells – illustrator extraordinaire

CONTENTS

Accept your role as an athlete
and realize the benefits of a
finely tuned body and mind.
Enjoy life and competition
in good health.

TOM HOLMES

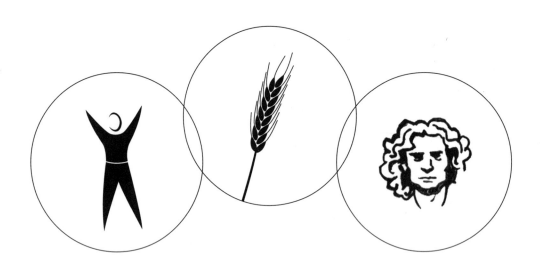

INTRODUCTION

WHAT DOES IT TAKE to be a successful competitive rider? Most experts agree it is a combination of desire, determination, focus, balance, flexibility, muscle awareness, and muscular endurance, to list a few qualities. Traditionally, riding skills have been developed through long hours of training in the saddle, a proven formula for which there is no substitute. This fact still remains true: If you want to be a successful rider, you must train hard and intelligently in the saddle. This is the foundation upon which winning is built. However, intensive riding is not all you can do to become a better rider.

By improving your physical and mental fitness you can utilize more of your full athletic potential to further develop your riding skills and competitiveness. A holistic and comprehensive fitness program can enhance your existing riding abilities. Achieving a higher degree of fitness will make your reactions quicker and your cues more precise. It will improve your balance, flexibility, and muscular endurance. By expanding your athletic potential you will ride with new confidence and authority.

The New Total Rider combines exercise, health, and nutrition principles into a balanced and integrated fitness program designed to complement your riding program. It is the result of a cooperative effort utilizing the expertise of health and fitness specialist and equestrian Barbara J. Beck, Ph.D., exercise physiologist Kay Roth, Ph.D., kinesiologist Bob Culver, nutrition and Ayurvedic expert Pilar Gutierrez Martin, renowned equine-sports psychologist Dr. Margot Nacey, and numerous other exercise professionals and world-class equestrians (see Acknowledgments, page iii). A cross-section of highly respected trainers and riders throughout the United States were studied and certain physical and mental qualities were found to be essential in developing the "ideal" rider in ten riding disciplines: dressage, hunt seat, cross-country and stadium jumping, reining, gymkhana, saddleseat, sidesaddle, and english and western pleasure. A blend of new and traditional exercises was then formulated to enhance these positive qualities. This became the fitness program known as The Equestrian Workout.

In **The New Total Rider**, the fitness program is integrated with effective health and nutritional guidelines to maximize your fitness benefits, and a powerful mental practice program to help you get the most out of your skills. All of the physical and mental exercises are intended to supplement your current riding program, and can be performed in the home, gym, or barn. **The New Total Rider** is divided into three parts:

▎ The Equestrian Workout targets your balance, flexibility, posture, muscular endurance, strength, and muscle awareness. These attributes are instrumental in developing a successful seat for riding regardless of your style.

▎ The Nutrition Advantage offers the latest in nutrition information. It will help you formulate a healthy diet that will increase and stabilize your energy levels throughout the day. With the right nutrition strategy, you will fatigue less easily, maintain mental sharpness, and combined with consistent exercise, lower your body fat percentage.

▎ The Mental Advantage delivers proven mental relaxation, stress management, focusing, and visualization techniques developed by psychologist Dr. Margot Nacey that will put you on top of your mental game.

1

Incorporated into The Equestrian Workout and The Mental Advantage are relaxation techniques useful in relieving muscular tension associated with stress and injury.

It's important to note that the key to success in any exercise program is not the type of equipment you use, but the mental attitude and approach you maintain. Simply put, you must train smart in order to train successfully. So, before you begin your workout, let's discuss some important fitness principles that will guide you to a new level of health and fitness:

▌ Before you begin any exercise program, you should receive a complete physical checkup from your physician.

▌ Let's debunk the most common of all exercise myths: "No pain, no gain." This rule applies only to an elite class of athletes whose highly conditioned bodies are capable of pushing past the normal physical limits intended for the rest of us mortals. Unless you're a world-class marathon runner or Arnold Schwarzeneggar's heir apparent, the rule of thumb for you should be: If you feel pain… Stop! This refers specifically to a sharp, shooting pain, not the mild aching sensation you will experience during exercise as your muscles begin to tire, or the stiffness you will sometimes feel before your muscles are thoroughly warmed. Many people learn to enjoy this tired sensation as it leaves a nice, warm feeling in your muscles, elevates your spirits, and is your body's way of communication that you are working hard enough.

Your body is amazingly accurate in informing you of its needs, once you learn how to listen to your body and train instinctively. If your shoulders are overworked, then rest them that day and exercise other areas of your body. If you feel that certain muscles are already highly developed, then concentrate more on weaker muscles, so you can ultimately achieve a balanced level of conditioning throughout your body.

▌ For any fitness program to be fully productive, you must combine three factors:

Exercise + Nutrition + Rest

It is this combination that will enable you to gain the most from your efforts by increasing the efficiency and quality of your exercises. Proper nutrition gives your muscle cells the nutrients they need to sustain exercise, and to recover and grow. Rest is critical for your muscles to have time to recover before you stress them again in your next workout, thus keeping the quality of each workout high and promoting maximum toning. You do not have to rest from your daily riding routine to compensate for added exercise. A good rule of thumb for insuring adequate rest is 48 hours between strenuous workouts. It is also wise to take a full week off from heavy exercise every 8 to 10 weeks to thoroughly rest your body and to prevent overtraining.

▌ Perhaps the most effective method to increase the quality of your exercise is to maximize every repetition by mentally focusing on the primary muscle as it is being worked. Concentrate on the sensation in the muscle as it contracts and extends, and maintain continuous tension in a slow and deliberate manner throughout the entire range of motion. This requires good form and slow, smooth movements. The idea is not to do as many repetitions as you can, but to make your muscles work as hard as possible in each individual rep. In the end, you will complete fewer reps, but you will produce better results, and maximizing results is your primary goal in any exercise program, not merely counting repetitions or minutes.

■ Always attempt to use good form and keep your movements smooth and deliberate; never jerk or bounce as this is very inefficient and may lead to injury.

■ Drink plenty of water during and after exercise. This prevents dehydration, and assists in flushing toxins/wastes produced by your muscle cells during exercise out of your body.

■ Vary your exercise routine to avoid boredom. You don't have to change the entire program; one or two exercises is sufficient to keep you fresh and looking forward to your next workout.

■ Loosen up and have fun with your fitness program. Take a bike ride, go swimming or cross-country skiing, or devise a game at home or at the barn. Turn on the stereo and work out with your spouse or several friends. You'll have more fun, and you'll discover a wonderful new source of motivation. Fitness should not only increase your riding skills and your capacity to enjoy life, but should be enjoyable itself.

■ Exercising will improve your muscle awareness, which will enable you to be more precise and knowledgeable in your movements in the saddle.

■ Remember that the exercises in The Equestrian Workout section are designed to enhance your current riding program and are not a substitute for training in the saddle.

3

10 REASONS TO EXERCISE

1. **Exercise improves the quality of your life.**
   The old adage, "Add life to your years, as well as years to your life by exercise" has considerable merit. A properly designed exercise program will give you more energy to do the activities you enjoy.

2. **Exercise relieves depression.**
   In her book, **Mental Skills for Physical People**, Dr. Dorothy V. Harris concluded that, "exercise is nature's best tranquilizer." Researchers have found, for example, that mildly to moderately depressed individuals who engage in aerobic exercise 15–30 minutes a day at least every other day typically experience a positive mood swing in two to three weeks.

3. **Exercise prevents certain types of cancer.**
   Studies have found that men and women who exercise are less likely to get colon cancer. Research has also suggested that women who do not exercise have more than two-and-one-half times the risk of developing cancer of the reproductive system and almost twice the chance of getting breast cancer.

4. **Exercise enhances your self-image.**
   Research has documented the assertion that individuals who exercise regularly feel better about themselves than sedentary individuals.

5. **Exercise relieves stress and anxiety.**
   Exercise dissipates those hormones and other chemicals which build up during periods of high stress. Exercise also generates a period of substantial emotional and physical relaxation that sets in approximately an hour-and-a-half after an intense workout.

6. **Exercise reduces the risk of heart disease.**
   Experts have found that non-exercisers have twice the risk of developing heart disease than individuals who exercise regularly.

7. **Exercise slows the aging process.**
   Proper exercise can increase your aerobic capacity as you get older, instead of losing aerobic fitness, as older people often do at the typical rate of ten percent per year. Past the age of thirty, you can actually become more aerobically fit if you exercise. Exercise can also result in better skin tone and muscle tone.

8. **Exercise increases the good (HDL) cholesterol.**
   Exercise is one of the few voluntary activities that is effective in raising your level of HDL—the type of cholesterol that lowers your risk of heart disease.

9. **Exercise improves the quality of sleep.**
   Researchers have found that exercisers go to sleep more quickly, sleep more soundly and are more refreshed than individuals who do not exercise.

10. **Exercise improves mental sharpness.**
    Numerous studies have shown that individuals who exercise regularly have better memories, better reaction times, and better concentration than non-exercisers.

Reprinted from the *Stairmaster Wellness Newsletter*, Vol. I, Iss. 1; written by Dr. James A. Peterson and Dr. Cedric X. Bryant; used by permission of Stairmaster Sports/Medical Products, Inc.

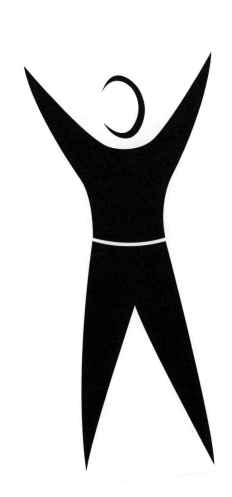

THE *NEW* TOTAL RIDER

1

The Equestrian Workout

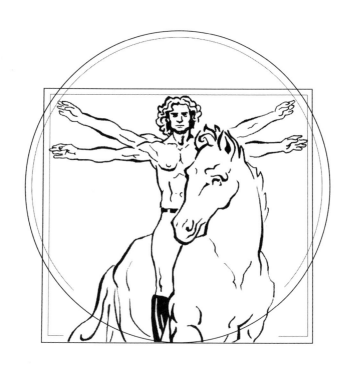

THE EQUESTRIAN WORKOUT

THE EXERCISES IN THE EQUESTRIAN WORKOUT are divided into three general categories:

1. **Strength and Muscular Endurance Exercises.** These exercises also include good hands and seat specific exercises.

2. **Flexibility, Posture and Balance Exercises.** These exercises are designed as a key part of your regular workout, and you can use them to stretch out before riding.

3. **Aerobic and Cardiovascular Exercises.**

Read through the following sections and familiarize yourself with the exercises. Then take a look at the suggested workouts for 30, 45 or 60 minutes; they are designed to provide a balanced workout that can fit the time you have available. The suggested workout schedule is 3 days a week with rest days in between each workout. Here's an example:

Exercise Schedule

Monday	Work out for 45 minutes
Tuesday	Rest
Wednesday	Work out for 45 minutes
Thursday	Rest
Friday	Work out for 45 minutes
Saturday	Rest
Sunday	Rest

The exercises are also designated as universal, beginner, intermediate and advanced, so you can choose the right exercises for your fitness level. Look to the title bar at the top of each page for that exercise's level of difficulty.

Universal exercises are for individuals of all fitness levels. You can increase the difficulty of these exercises by raising the number of repetitions, or by adding weight or resistance.

■ **Beginner** exercises are designed for the individual starting a fitness program for the first time or resuming one after a prolonged period of reduced activity. **All** readers, regardless of their fitness level, should start with the beginner exercises, then progress slowly to the more challenging levels.

■ **Intermediate** exercises are for the individual who has comfortably completed the beginner levels and is ready for a higher degree of difficulty.

■ **Advanced** exercises are for the person who has comfortably completed the intermediate level exercises and is ready for a greater challenge.

■ **Alternate** exercises have been included to provide a little variety to help you stay motivated. Where applicable, choose the one that most appeals to you and try it out.

Remember that exercise is only as effective as you make it. You can experience substantial benefits from your workout if you exercise intelligently, and stay motivated, focused and precise in form. Here are some helpful tips on exercising wisely:

■ Always begin your workout with a warm-up.

■ Perform each exercise in a smooth and controlled manner. Quick, jerky movements decrease the efficiency of the exercise and often lead to injury.

■ Exercise requires mental focus. Carefully read your instructions and focus on your form throughout every single repetition. Precise form creates maximum efficiency and pays off with superior results.

■ Ensure that you are well hydrated before your workout. Take frequent sips of water during your workout to stay hydrated and stabilize your energy level. Don't wait until you are noticeably thirsty: by then your energy level has already dropped.

▌ Move quickly (30–60 seconds) between each exercise. However, it's okay if you need to take more time and rest.

▌ Exercise with a partner if possible. A good exercise partner will provide support, motivation, help you monitor your form, and enable you to get more oomph out of your workout.

▌ See a fitness professional before starting any exercise program. If you experience any pain or injury, do not self-medicate, see a medical professional immediately.

For many people, time constraints are a real problem. If you don't have the time to perform the entire exercise program then do what you can. Each exercise, if done well, will help improve your fitness level and riding skill.

Exercise is enjoyable and rewarding, so have some fun with it!

WARM-UP

YOUR WORKOUT SHOULD ALWAYS BEGIN with a gradual warm-up. Why is a warm-up so important? Its purpose is to elevate your deep muscle and overall body temperatures in preparation for all the stretching and contracting your muscles and other soft tissues will experience. More specifically, a thorough warm-up will:

▮ Lessen the potential for injury during exercising and stretching. When you stretch a cold muscle, you risk tearing muscle fibers and their tendinous attachments.

▮ Reduce muscle soreness.

▮ Speed up your metabolism and nerve impulse transmissions, and increase your blood flow and oxygen supply, which will result in improved performance and physical working capacity during exercise.

Here are some warm-up guidelines:

▮ Begin with an easy range of motion and intensity, and then gradually increase to a moderate range of motion and intensity.

▮ You are warm enough when you begin to sweat after at least 10 minutes of continuous warm-up.

▮ No more than 10 minutes should elapse from the end of your warm-up and the beginning of your exercises or activity.

A warm-up can be performed almost anywhere. It can be any moderate activity that sufficiently raises your body temperature and causes you to sweat. Here are 3 excellent outdoor warm-up activities:

▮ A moderate-brisk walk for 10–15 minutes.

▮ A moderate bike ride for 10–15 minutes.

▮ Lead your horse on a moderate-brisk walk for 10–15 minutes.

If the weather isn't to your liking or you just don't want to venture outside, this simple, all-weather warm-up will get you primed for your workout:

▮ Begin by walking in place with your arms down at your sides. After 1 minute, begin raising your knees higher and slowly swinging your arms front to back in unison with your steps. Start with small movements and gradually increase to larger movements. To add a little variety try the following variations:

▮ Raise your arms above your head in time with your steps.

▮ Extend your arms out to the sides in time with your steps.

▮ Extend your arms in front of your body in time with your steps.

▮ Step heel in front and toe in back.

▮ Dance and sing. You can amaze your friends with your stylistic interpretations.

If you have surpassed 10 minutes and you are sweating, then you have successfully raised your body and muscle temperatures to the desired level. So stop singing and begin your exercising and stretching as soon as possible (within 10 minutes ... tops).

Flex-Sets

Flex-Sets are easier to perform than they are to say. Instead of standing around while you rest between exercise sets, alternate your strength/muscular endurance set with 10 seconds of mild stretching on the same muscle group. For example, immediately after you've completed a set of Wall Squats, do a mild to moderate Quad Stretch for 10 seconds. This will help you maintain your flexibility while you build and tone muscle. If you're not sure which stretch to perform, then consult the Muscle Reference Guide following.

MUSCLE REFERENCE GUIDE

MUSCLES	STRENGTH & MUSCULAR ENDURANCE	FLEXIBILITY & POSTURE
Abdominals	Crunches 5-Way Crunches Hard Rocks Oblique Curl	Ventral Stretch
Lower Back	The Pointer Prone Trunk Extension The Advanced Pointer	Dorsal Flex Angry Cat & Sway-Back Horse Cross-legged Bow Ventral Stretch
Inner Thighs	Adductor Lift The Squeeze Adductor-Quad Sets	Sumo Stretch Adductor Stretch
Quadriceps-Psoas	Quad-Psoas Lift	
Quadriceps	Wall Squats	Quad Stretch
Gluteals	Glute-Hamstring Lift	Dorsal Flex Cross-legged Bow Hip Stretch
Hamstrings	Hamstring Curl Supine Leg Curl	Seated Ham Stretch Standing Ham Stretch
Calves	Heel Raise	Push-The-Wall-Down Soleus Stretch
Chest	Wall Pushes Kneeling Push-Ups Push-Ups	Doorway Stretch 7th Inning Stretch
Upper back & shoulders	Theraband Flye Prone Flye	Cross-legged Bow
Shoulders	Forward Arm Raise Lateral Arm Raise	
Triceps	Kickbacks Overhead Extensions	
Biceps	Rotation Curl Hammer Curl	
Wrist Extensors	Wrist Swing	Steeple (for dexterity)
Wrist Flexors	Orange Crush	

12

STRENGTH & MUSCULAR ENDURANCE EXERCISES

Muscular endurance refers to your muscle's ability to contact repeatedly against resistance. Any improvement in muscular endurance is closely connected with improvement in strength and maintenance of a certain degree of flexibility. As your strength increases, so does your muscular endurance, as long as your muscle in moving within your comfortable range of motion. As a rider-athlete, you can benefit from this training in a number of ways:

▐ It will strengthen your muscles, tendons, ligaments, joint capsules and even your bones. These will increase in density and become more resistant to injury.

▐ It will enable you to work/play harder and longer without experiencing debilitating muscle fatigue.

▐ It will improve your muscle coordination, muscle awareness and agility, which will help you become more precise in the saddle and enhance your riding appearance. Agility is your ability to make a quick and coordinated change in direction. It is crucial to any successful athletic performance and it can help you avoid potential accident and injury.

▐ Strength and muscular endurance will positively enhance your stretching program and your dynamic flexibility.

These exercises are not designed to dramatically increase your muscle size. They work primarily to improve the efficiency of your muscle fibers. Through consistent and correct use of these exercises, your muscles will show increased tone and definition.

Note: Consider this possible riding scenario. You're in temporary disagreement with your horse, yet due to your improved physical capabilities, you're able to gracefully maintain your balance, stylishly retain your composure and instantly regain your seat. Needless to say, you successfully avoid unscheduled contact with the ground.

Here are a few guidelines for safe and efficient strength and muscular endurance training:

▐ Take it slow and easy for the first week if you are performing these exercises for the first time or after a layoff of 2 weeks or more. Avoid unnecessary extreme soreness and allow your body sufficient time to adjust before you raise your intensity level.

▐ Expect mild soreness to occur when you begin exercising and any time you increase your intensity. This is okay. You will eventually begin to enjoy this sensation … seriously, it could happen.

▐ Follow all exercise instructions precisely.

▐ Your movements during exercise should be smooth and controlled. Jerking and bouncing movements are very inefficient and can cause injury.

▐ Drink sips of water throughout your workout to avoid dehydration and to help maintain a high energy level.

▐ Get the most out of each exercise by focusing on your primary muscles during every single repetition and by making those muscles work as hard as possible. This is how you successfully raise your intensity.

▐ Move quickly from one exercise set into your stretch and then into your next exercise set for maximum fitness benefit. Take more time if needed.

13

Good Hands Exercises

The Good Hands exercises are designed to help you ride with softer and more precise hands by improving the dexterity, muscular endurance and strength in your fingers and forearms.

Seat Specific Exercises

Choose the appropriate exercise for your style of riding and add it to your workout:

▌ Forward Seat – hunter, jumper, english pleasure, etc.

▌ Balanced Seat – dressage, western, gymkhana, etc.

▌ Saddleseat

CRUNCHES

HOW IMPORTANT IS DEVELOPING strong abdominal muscles to your overall fitness and to you as an equestrian-athlete?

Answer: Your abdominals are engaged in nearly every movement you make. They enable you to flex forward at the waist, to twist at the waist, to stabilize your "trunk", and to use your arms and legs in independent and coordinated movements. Weak abdominal muscles contribute to poor balance and agility and to the development of chronic lower back problems.

Conclusion: You need all of the abdominal strength you can get ... so start crunching. Crunches are a good exercise for the prevention of lower back pain and injury.

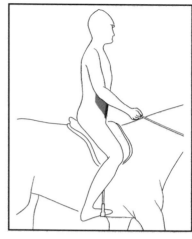

primary muscles

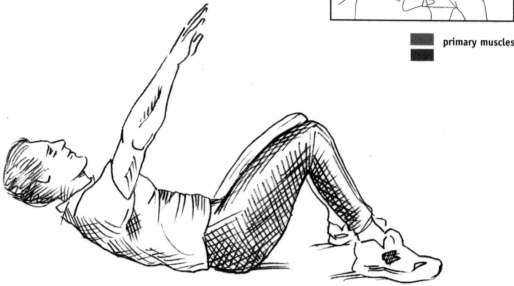

■ Lie on your back with your feet flat on the floor and your knees bent at an angle sharper than 90 degrees.

■ Point your hands above your knees at a 60° angle.

■ Follow your hands with your eyes and gently point your jaw. This will place your head in a neutral position and reduce the amount of stress on your neck.

■ Press your lower back to the ground, then squeeze your abdominal muscles and lift your upper body toward the sky until your shoulder blades are off the floor.

■ Exhale as you crunch ... allow your con-

tracting abdominal muscles and diaphragm to push your breath out.

■ Hold for 1 second.

■ Inhaling softly, slowly lower your upper body until your shoulder blades touch the floor to complete one repetition.

■ Repeat until you reach fatigue.

■ This will complete 1 set

■ Perform a total of 2 sets.

FLEX-SET

Perform the Ventral Stretch for 10 seconds immediately after each set of Crunches.

15

5-WAY CRUNCHES

ONE

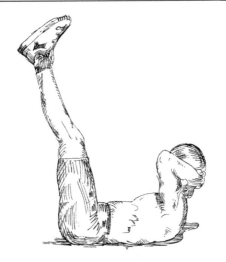

▌ Lie on your back with your legs extended together straight up into the air.

▌ Clasp your hands behind your neck.

▌ Slowly lift your upper body toward the sky, exhaling softly as you lift. Remember not to pull your neck up with your arms.

▌ Hold for a count of 1 second, then inhaling, lower yourself until your shoulder blades touch the floor. This completes 1 repetition.

▌ Perform 10–15 repetitions.

TWO

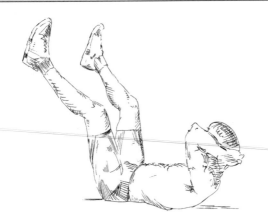

▌ Without pausing, spread your feet apart in the air and perform 10–15 more repetitions.

THREE

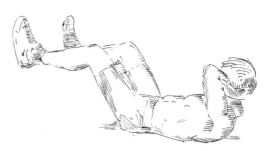

▌ Without pausing, bend your knees 90 degrees (your legs are still apart) and perform 10–15 more repetitions.

FOUR

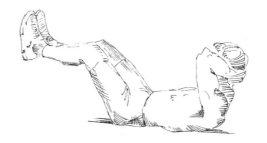

▌ Without pausing, bring your knees together and perform 10–15 more repetitions.

FIVE

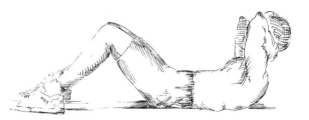

▌ Without pausing, lower your feet to the floor with your knees still bent and perform 10–15 final repetitions.

FLEX-SET

Perform the Ventral Stretch for 10 seconds immediately after each set of 5-Way Crunches.

HARD ROCKS

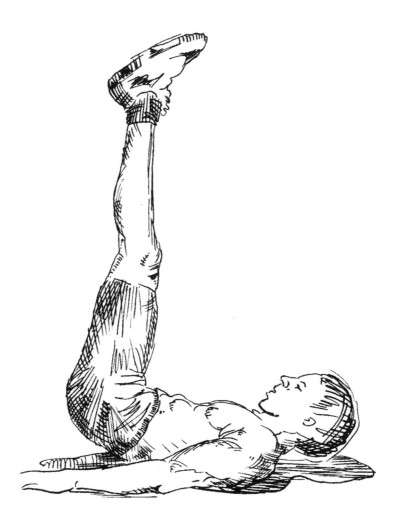

ONCE YOU ARE CAPABLE of performing the advanced-level abdominal exercises, add the Hard Rocks to your routine and perform in addition to the 5-Way Crunches and the Intermediate-Advanced Oblique Curl.

▌ Lie on your back and place your hands palms down under your hips. Your head should be lifted off of the floor (Use a large pillow for support if your neck fatigues easily).

▌ Extend your legs straight up in the air.

▌ Exhaling softly, squeeze your abdominal muscles and push your hips and legs 4-6 inches higher in the air.

▌ Hold for 1 second then return to the start position as you inhale.

▌ Repeat until fatigued.

FLEX-SET

Perform the Ventral Stretch for 10 seconds immediately after each set of Hard Rocks.

OBLIQUE CURL

Your obliques enable you to rotate at the waist and to pull (flex) yourself up when you are behind vertical in a sitting position. This is critical to your ability as a rider to maintain balance in the saddle.

Your obliques also (along with your other abdominal muscles) help stabilize your pelvis, which enables you to maintain good posture. An additional benefit is that tight obliques contribute to the appearance of a trim waist. The Oblique Curl is a good exercise for the prevention of lower back pain.

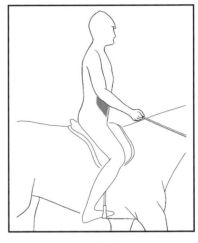

primary muscles

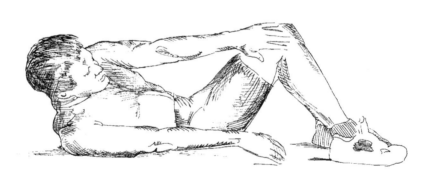

- Lie on your back with your feet flat on the floor and your knees bent at an angle sharper than 90 degrees.

- Point your hands above your knees.

- Exhaling softly, slowly curl up (twisting slightly counter-clockwise and squeezing those oblique muscles) and extend your right hand past your left knee until your shoulder blades are off the floor.

- Reach behind your head with one hand if you want more support for your neck.

- Lower yourself (inhaling softly) until your shoulder blades touch the floor.

- This completes 1 repetition.

- Repeat until you reach fatigue.

- Repeat exercise with your left hand extending past your right knee.

- This completes 1 set.

- Perform 2 sets.

FLEX-SET

Perform the Ventral Stretch for 10 seconds immediately after each set of Oblique Curl.

THE POINTER

BEGINNER

PROJECTIONS SHOW THAT 92% OF AMERICANS are destined to suffer from chronic back pain. Soreness in the lower back also ranks as the most common complaint among riders. Your lower back muscles work continuously during riding to stabilize your upper body and absorb the natural concussions created by your horse in motion. The facts reveal that the majority of "bad backs" are caused by poor posture, weak lower back muscles, and weak abdominal muscles. Fortunately, relief for these back problems can be attained through sensible exercise. The Pointer will strengthen your back muscles and hip flexors, improve your balance, and enhance your muscle awareness. This will eventually enable you to maintain a proper riding position longer without experiencing lower back strain and soreness. It may also keep you from becoming another "bad-back" statistic.

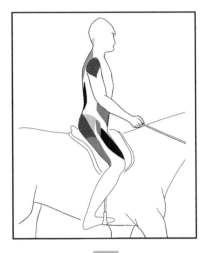

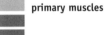
primary muscles

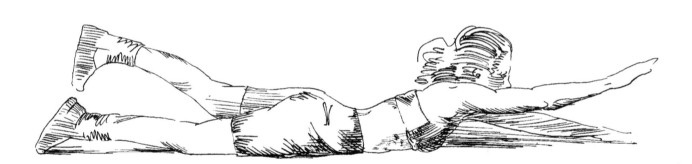

■ Lie on your front with your arms and legs extended.

■ Slowly raise your left arm and right leg as high as is comfortable. It should take a count of 10 seconds to raise your arm and leg.

■ Breathe normally and hold this position for a minimum of 15 seconds.

■ Slowly lower your arm and leg (for a count of 10) to the floor.

■ Repeat steps 1 and 2 with your opposite arm and leg. This completes 1 repetition.

■ Perform a minimum of 3–5 repetitions per set.

■ Perform 2 sets.

19

FLEX-SET

Perform the Dorsal Flex for 10 seconds immediately after each set of The Pointer.

PRONE TRUNK EXTENSION

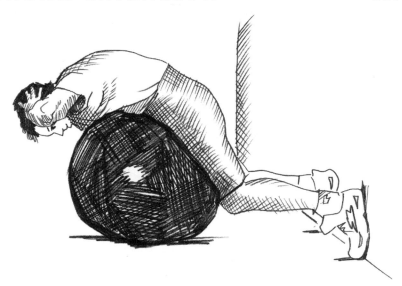

▌ Lie face down on the ball with your knees bent and feet pressed against the wall.

▌ Clasp your hands behind your neck.

▌ Squeeze your abdominals and glutes.

▌ Slowly raise your chest until your spine is straight or slightly extended. Keep squeezing your abs.

▌ Return to start and repeat until fatigued.

▌ Perform 2 sets.

▌ To raise the intensity level, try these two variations:

1. Place your hands on your forehead or your fists at your temples.

2. For an advanced exercise, perform back extension, hold and perform back flye.

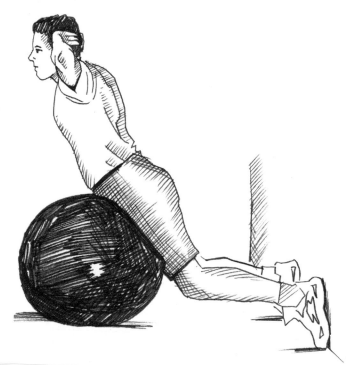

FLEX-SET

Perform the Dorsal Flex for 10 seconds immediately after each set of Prone Trunk Extension.

ADVANCED POINTER

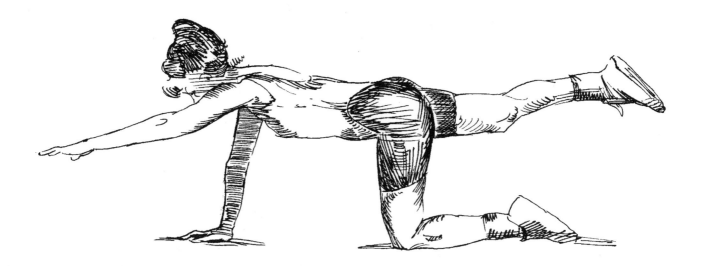

- Lower yourself onto all fours, placing your hands and your knees shoulder-width apart.

- Face the floor and hold your back in a flat position (neither swayed nor arched) by tightening your abdominal and lower back muscles. This places your back in a safe "neutral" position and increases the efficiency of the exercise.

- Slowly raise your left arm and right leg for a count of 10 seconds until both are fully extended and parallel to the floor. Breathe normally and maintain this position for a minimum of 15 seconds.

- Slowly lower (for a count of 10) your arm and leg to the floor.

- Repeat with your opposite arm and leg. This completes 1 repetition.

- Perform a minimum of 3–5 repetitions per set. To increase difficulty, you can perform additional repetitions, wear ankle weights, riding boots, or ski boots, etc.

- Perform 2 sets.

21

FLEX-SET

Perform the Dorsal Flex for 10 seconds immediately after each set of The Advanced Pointer.

ADDUCTOR LIFT

I**N THE FORWARD SEAT**, your adductors are used in cueing and collecting your horse, forming the primary basis for support. In balanced set, your adductors are used independently to cue and to stabilize your upper and lower body. Regardless of your riding style and degree of fitness you will need to strengthen your adductors in order to physically improve as a rider. The Adductor Lift is designed to build strength and muscular endurance in your inner thighs.

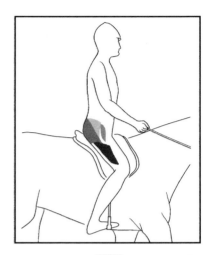

primary muscles

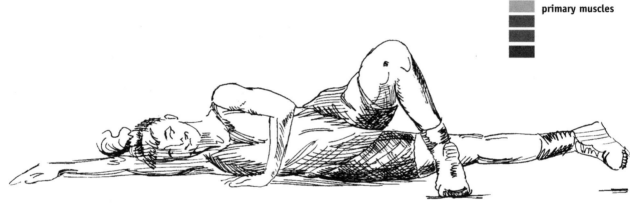

- Lie on your right side with your legs straight and your head supported by your extended right arm.

- Place your left hand flat on the floor in front of your chest for balance.

- Cross your upper leg over your extended lower leg and place your foot flat on the floor.

- Slowly raise your lower (right) leg a comfortable distance off the floor—this may be only a few inches. Breath normally and hold for a count of 3 seconds. Keep your body straight, do not bend at the hips.

- Finish the lift by slowly lowering your leg in a smooth and controlled manner.

- Repeat until you reach fatigue.

- Switch sides and perform exercise with your left leg for an equal number of repetitions. This completes 1 set.

- To increase difficulty, perform additional repetitions, wear ankle weights, riding boots, or ski boots, etc.

- Perform 2 sets.

FLEX-SET

Perform the Sumo Stretch for 10 seconds immediately after each set of Adductor Lift.

THE SQUEEZE

UNIVERSAL

THE SQUEEZE ALSO BUILDS STRENGTH and muscular endurance in your adductor muscles. Why have 2 exercises for the same muscle group? Because our riding instructors are always instructing us to drop our stirrups and ride in a 2-point position for what seems an eternity. Instructors are never satisfied … and with good reason. Few riders are gifted with sufficient strength and muscular endurance in their adductors.

To perform The Squeeze you will need a basketball, volleyball, or soccer ball. The secret to this exercise is to underinflate the ball slightly so it gives a little. This will increase your comfort and efficiency.

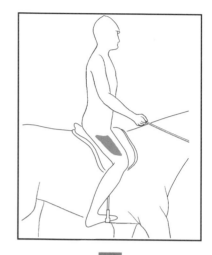

primary muscles

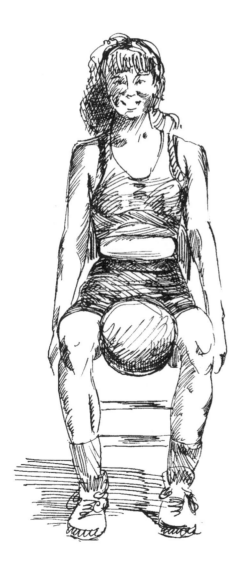

❚ Sit in a chair with your feet shoulder-width apart.

❚ Place a ball (basketball, volleyball, soccer ball, etc.) between your legs just above the knees.

❚ Squeeze and hold for 7 seconds.

❚ Relax for 3 seconds.

❚ Repeat for a minimum of 10 repetitions or until fatigued.

❚ Perform 2 sets.

You can also perform this exercise standing with your knees bent, squeezing a large pillow, or sitting in a saddle on a saddle rack.

23

FLEX-SET

Perform the Sumo Stretch for 10 seconds immediately after each set of The Squeeze.

ADDUCTOR QUAD SETS

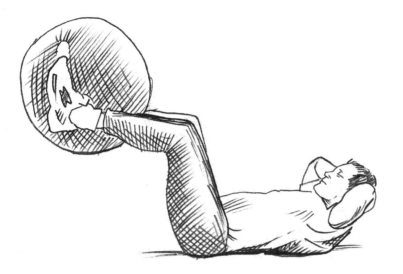

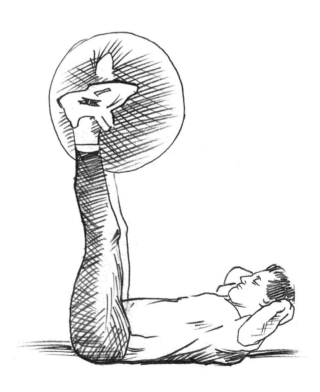

■ Lie on your back with ball centered between your feet with your hips and knees at 90 degree angles.

■ Squeeze the ball between your feet as hard as you can.

■ Slowly straighten your legs toward the sky, maintaining 90 degree hip angle. Exhale as you extend your legs.

■ Keep squeezing.

■ Return to start position.

■ Repeat until fatigued.

■ Perform 2 sets.

■ For a more difficult challenge, try adding this variation: When your legs are extended toward the sky, press your lower back into the floor and lift your hips off the ground.

FLEX-SET

Perform the Sumo Stretch for 10 seconds immediately after each set of Adductor-Quad Sets.

QUAD-PSOAS LIFT

Y OUR QUADRICEPS ENABLE YOU to extend your legs at the knees, making them the antagonistic muscles to your hamstrings … as one muscle contracts the other relaxes and lengthens. Like the hamstrings, your quadriceps allow you to walk and run, to mount and dismount, to keep your legs in a correct fore-hind riding position, and to post the trot. The quad lift will build strength and muscular endurance in your quadriceps. You'll have to excuse the nagging … but remember to always exercise your quadriceps and hamstrings equally so that one doesn't become stronger than the other.

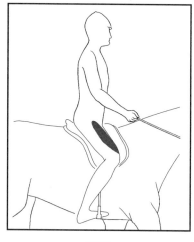

primary muscles

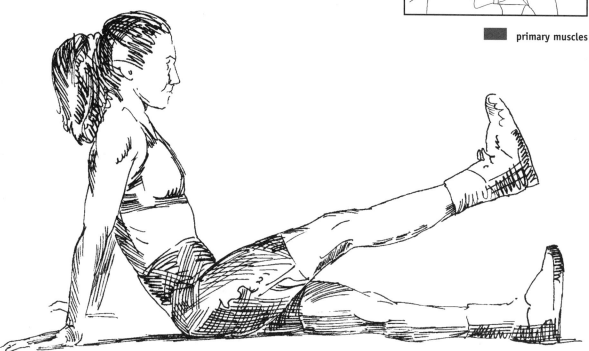

■ Sit on the floor with your legs extended in front of you. Support yourself with your hands slightly behind you on the floor.

■ Breathe normally and slowly raise your right leg 8–14 inches above the floor with your toes pointing skyward. Focus on squeezing your quadriceps muscle as you lift.

■ Hold for 1–3 seconds then lower.

■ Repeat with your left leg for an equal number of repetitions. This completes 1 set.

■ To increase the difficulty of this exercise, perform additional repetitions, wear ankle weights, riding boots, or ski boots, etc.

■ Perform 2 sets.

25

FLEX-SET

Perform the Quad Stretch for 10 seconds immediately after each set of Quad-Psoas Lift.

WALL SQUATS

UNIVERSAL

primary muscles:
gluteus maximus
hamstrings
quadriceps

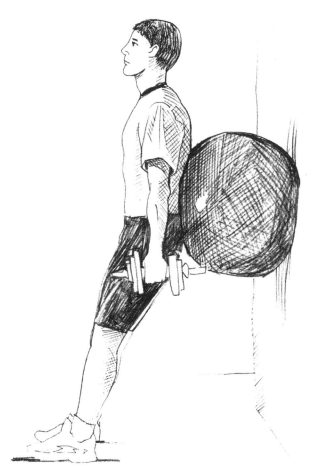

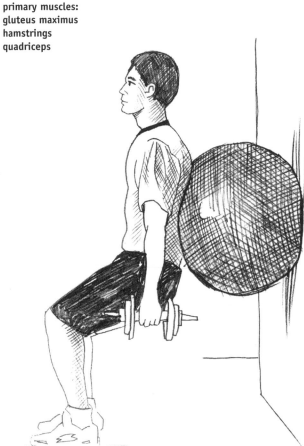

- Stand with the Swiss ball between your lower back and the wall. Walk your feet forward 6–12 inches and keep them shoulder width apart. This will cause you to lean slightly on the ball.

- Point your arms directly in front of your chest for balance.

- Bend your knees and lower yourself as far as you can without lifting your heels off the floor (Don't go lower than a 90 degree bend in your knees … any lower will stress your knees).

- Hold for 1 second. Look straight ahead and focus on your quadriceps as you exercise. Do not fully straighten your legs when you return to the start position.

- Inhale as you lower your body and exhale as you return to standing.

- Repeat for a minimum of 20 repetitions or until fatigued. Shoot for 100 repetitions.

- Perform 2 sets.

- To increase difficulty, perform exercise with 2 dumbbells of at least 10 lbs.

- You can also increase the intensity by squeezing a small volleyball, etc. between your knees.

FLEX-SET

Perform the Quad Stretch for 10 seconds immediately after each set of Wall Squats.

26

GLUTE-HAMSTRING LIFT

Y OUR HAMSTRINGS FLEX YOUR LEGS at the knees enabling you to walk, run, and sit. Hamstrings play more of a secondary role in riding. They help you mount and dismount your horse, maintain correct leg position in the saddle, and post the trot. The Hamstring Lift will improve your strength and muscular endurance and maintain critical muscle balance in your legs (combined with the Quad Lift) .

What is "muscle balance" and why is it a big deal? Antagonistic muscles such as your hamstrings and quadriceps need to be equivalent in strength for you to maintain healthy joints. For example, if your hamstring is stronger than your quadriceps (or vice-versa), then your knee is pulled out of its natural alignment making it more vulnerable to injury and chronic problems.

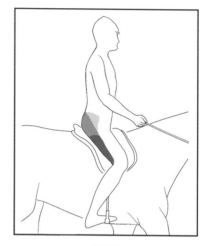

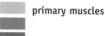

primary muscles

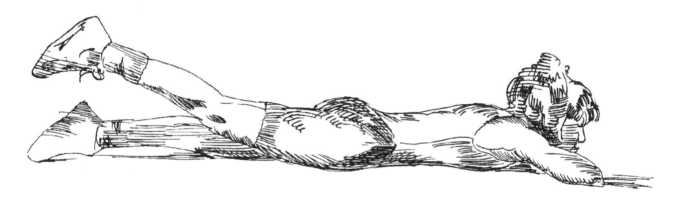

▌ Lie on your front with your legs extended and your chin resting on your hands.

▌ Raise your right leg 1 foot off the floor.

▌ Hold for 1–3 seconds. Breathe normally throughout the entire exercise.

▌ Relax. It is important to keep your hips firmly on the floor as you perform this exercise.

▌ Repeat until fatigued.

▌ Repeat exercise with your left leg for an equal number of repetitions. This completes 1 set.

▌ To increase the difficulty of this exercise, perform additional repetitions, wear ankle weights, riding boots, or ski boots, etc.

▌ Perform a total of 2 sets.

27

FLEX-SET

Perform the Hip Stretch for 10 seconds immediately after each set of Glute-Hamstring Lift. Stretch both hips.

HAMSTRING CURL

Your hamstrings flex your legs at the knees enabling you to walk, run, and sit. Hamstrings play more of a secondary role in riding. They help you mount and dismount your horse, maintain correct leg position in the saddle, and post the trot. The Hamstring Lift will improve your strength and muscular endurance and maintain critical muscle balance in your legs (combined with the Quad Lift).

What is "muscle balance" and why is it a big deal? Antagonistic muscles such as your hamstrings and quadriceps need to be equivalent in strength for you to maintain healthy joints. For example, if your hamstring is stronger than your quadriceps (or vice-versa), then your knee is pulled out of its natural alignment making it more vulnerable to injury and chronic problems.

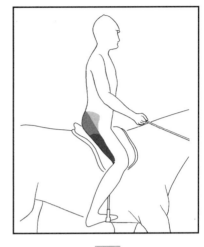

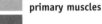 **primary muscles**

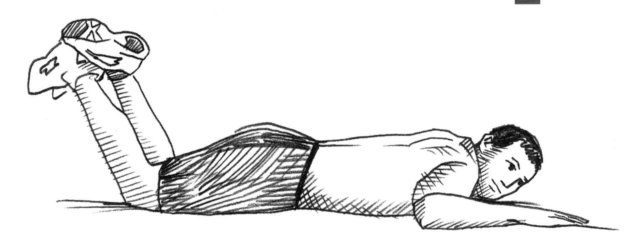

28

- Lie on your front with your legs extended and your chin resting on your hands.

- Place your left ankle over your right ankle.

- Using your left leg for resistance, bend your right knee as far as possible.

- Hold for 1 second. Breathe normally throughout the entire exercise.

- Relax. It is important to keep your hips firmly on the floor as you perform this exercise.

- Repeat until fatigued.

- Change legs and repeat exercise for an equal number of repetitions. This completes 1 set.

- Perform a total of 2 sets.

FLEX-SET

Perform the Standing Ham Stretch for 10 seconds immediately after each set of Hamstring Curl. Stretch both hamstrings.

SUPINE LEG CURL

YOUR HAMSTRINGS FLEX YOUR LEGS at the knees enabling you to walk, run, and sit. Hamstrings play more of a secondary role in riding. They help you mount and dismount your horse, maintain correct leg position in the saddle, and post the trot. The Hamstring Lift will improve your strength and muscular endurance and maintain critical muscle balance in your legs (combined with the Quad Lift).

What is "muscle balance" and why is it a big deal? Antagonistic muscles such as your hamstrings and quadriceps need to be equivalent in strength for you to maintain healthy joints. For example, if your hamstring is stronger than your quadriceps (or vice-versa), then your knee is pulled out of its natural alignment making it more vulnerable to injury and chronic problems.

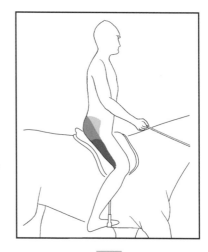

primary muscles

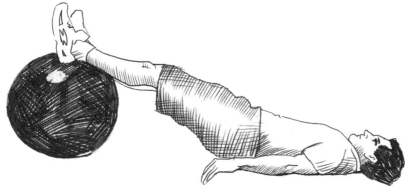

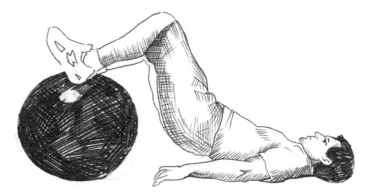

■ Lie on your back on the floor with your legs extended and the physio-ball under your ankles. Place your hands at your sides.

■ Press hips toward the sky 4–6 inches. Then draw your feet and the ball towards your buttocks.

■ Hold and squeeze hamstrings for 1 second.

■ Return to start position.

■ Perform a total of 2 sets.

■ To increase intensity, place hands across your chest.

FLEX-SET

Perform the Seated Ham Stretch for 10 seconds immediately after each set of Supine Leg Curl. Stretch both hamstrings.

HEEL RAISE

Tʜᴇ Hᴇᴇʟ Rᴀɪsᴇ ᴡɪʟʟ ʙᴜɪʟᴅ sᴛʀᴇɴɢᴛʜ and muscular endurance in your gastrocnemius and soleus muscles. Although calf-flexibility is more important to you as a rider-athlete, strength training is necessary to maintain adequate muscle balance in your legs. You will need to improvise a suitable step for this exercise. A set of stairs, a raised doorway, or any stable object that is at least 5 inches off the ground will suffice. You will also need a nearby wall or post to balance against.

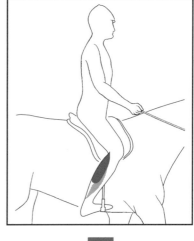

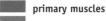
primary muscles

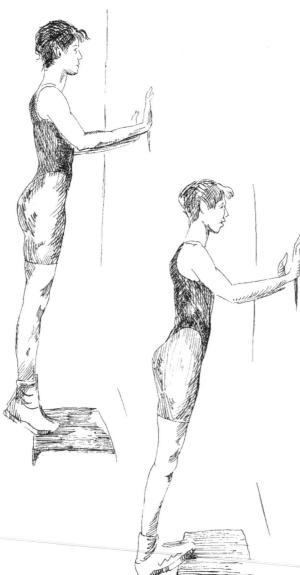

▌ Stand with the balls of your feet and your toes on the step, and balance yourself with your hands.

▌ Raise up on your toes as far as you can go.

▌ Breathe normally and hold for 1 second.

▌ Gently drop your heels as low as they will comfortably go.

▌ Hold for 1 second then raise your heels again. Focus on and squeeze your calf muscles as you raise and lower. Be sure that your movements are smooth and controlled.

▌ This completes 1 repetition.

▌ Repeat until fatigued.

▌ Perform 2 sets.

30

FLEX-SET

Perform Push-The-Wall-Down for 10 seconds immediately after each set of Heel Raise.

WALL PUSHES

Wall Pushes provide another ingredient in your posture building formula. Improving the strength in your pectoralis major will maintain adequate muscle balance with your upper back muscles. Secondary emphasis is placed on your triceps.

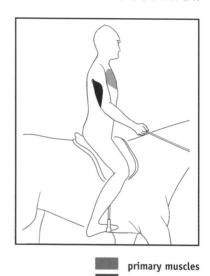

primary muscles

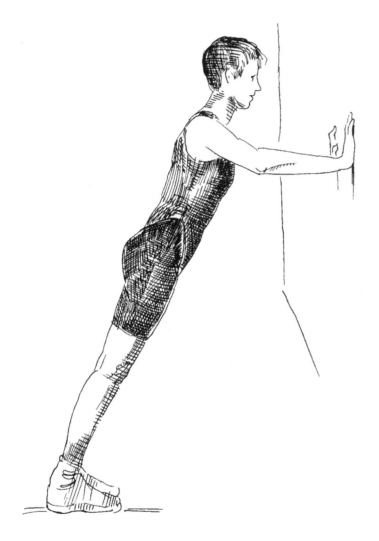

- Position yourself one and a half arms' length from a wall.

- Stand with your feet together, lean forward and place both hands chest high and shoulder width apart on the wall. Your elbows should be slightly bent.

- Bend your elbows and lean as far as you can into the wall. Breathe normally.

- Slowly push yourself away from the wall and back to the start position. Focus on and squeeze your chest muscles.

- Repeat for a minimum of 15 repetitions or until fatigued.

- Perform 2 sets.

FLEX-SET

Perform the 7th Inning Stretch for 10 seconds immediately after each set of Wall Pushes.

KNEELING PUSH-UPS

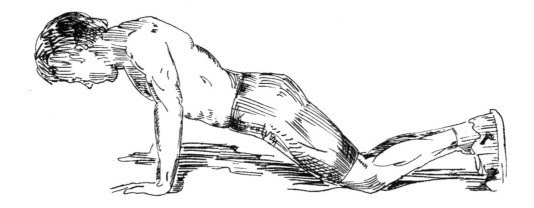

▌ Lower yourself onto your hands and knees with your hands shoulder-width apart.

▌ Bending at the elbows and inhaling softly, lower your upper body until your nose almost touches the floor.

▌ Keep your back straight.

▌ Hold for 1 second.

▌ Exhaling slowly, push yourself until your arms are almost fully extended.

▌ Repeat until fatigued.

▌ Perform 2 sets.

FLEX-SET

Perform the 7th Inning Stretch for 10 seconds immediately after each set of Kneeling Push-Ups.

PUSH-UPS

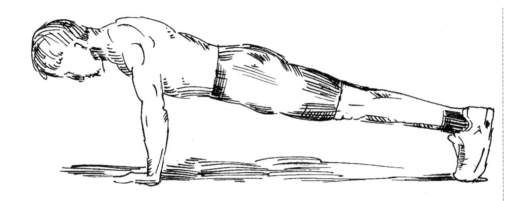

- Lie on your front with your legs extended and your hands shoulder-width apart on the floor.

- Exhaling slowly, push up onto your hands and toes until your arms are almost fully extended.

- Keep your back and legs straight.

- Hold for 1 second.

- Inhale softly, bend at the elbows and lower to an inch above the floor.

- Hold for 1 second then push up again.

- Repeat until fatigued.

- Perform 2 sets.

- To develop your balance, place the physio-ball under your thighs, knees or ankles. The exercise becomes harder as the ball moves closer to your feet.

FLEX-SET

Perform the 7th Inning Stretch for 10 seconds immediately after each set of Push-Ups.

RUBBERBAND FLYE

UNIVERSAL

Poor posture is a major problem among riders as well as the general public. Individuals in both cases subconsciously collapse their chests and round their shoulders. Bad posture in the saddle can cause poor balance, fatigue, and improper cueing. The major contributors to poor posture are laziness and weak back muscles which allow your chest and shoulders to roll forward. The Rubberband Flye addresses this problem by developing strength and muscular endurance in your trapezius and posterior deltoid muscles, and by laterally stretching your chest muscles. This will help you improve your posture and attain a taller riding position through increased upper body control and muscle awareness. You will also improve your overall balance by "pulling" your upper body into correct alignment with your lower body.

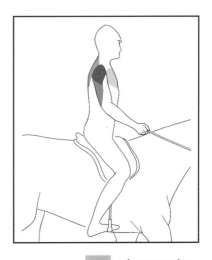

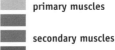

primary muscles

secondary muscles

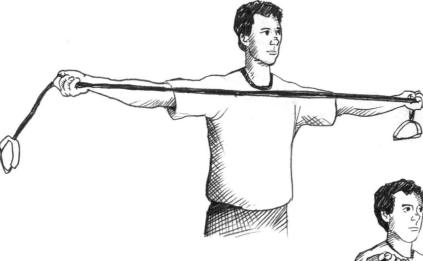

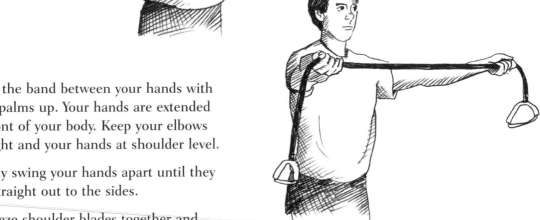

■ Hold the band between your hands with your palms up. Your hands are extended in front of your body. Keep your elbows straight and your hands at shoulder level.

■ Slowly swing your hands apart until they are straight out to the sides.

■ Squeeze shoulder blades together and hold for 1 second. Slowly return to front. Repeat until fatigued.

■ Perform 2 sets.

■ The closer your hands are together at the start position, the greater the intensity.

FLEX-SET

Perform Cross-legged Bow with your head dropped toward the floor for 10 seconds immediately after each set of Theraband Flye.

PRONE FLYE

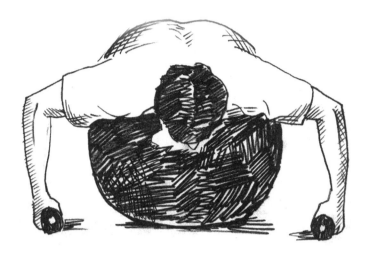

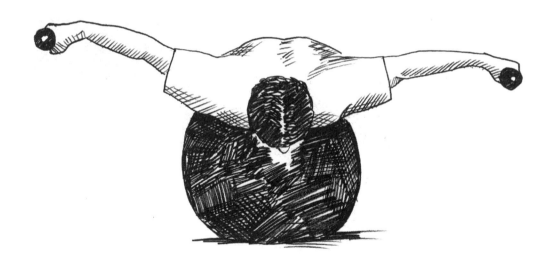

35

▌ Lie face down with the physio-ball under your abdomen and chest. Bend your elbows to 90 degrees and arms resting on the sides of the physio-ball.

▌ Slowly raise your elbows up to the level of your shoulders.

▌ Return to start. Repeat until fatigued.

▌ Perform 2 sets.

▌ To increase difficulty, perform exercise with light- to moderate-weight dumbbells.

FLEX-SET

Perform Cross-legged Bow with your head dropped toward the floor for 10 seconds immediately after each set of Prone Flye.

FORWARD ARM RAISE

Tʜᴇ Fᴏʀᴡᴀʀᴅ Aʀᴍ Rᴀɪsᴇ builds muscular endurance in your anterior deltoid which will benefit your posture and will help you avoid using your reins and your horse's mouth for support. But you never lean on your horse's mouth …. Are you sure, oh-leaden-armed-one? Many riders subconsciously rely on a little extra counter-tension in their reins to support their arms and shoulders.

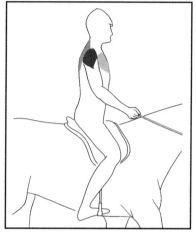

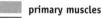

primary muscles

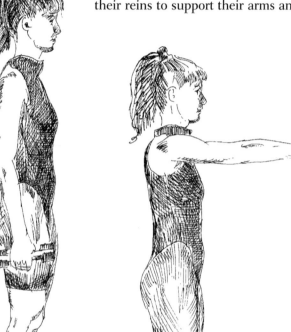

▌ You will need 2 small dumbbells for this exercise. They should be light enough for you to lift easily for the first few repetitions.

▌ Stand with your feet shoulder width apart and your knees slightly bent.

▌ Start with your hands down at your sides and your palms facing each other.

▌ Breathing normally, slowly raise your right arm until it is parallel to the floor. As you raise your arm, turn your hand counter-clockwise (supinate) until your palm faces the floor).

▌ Hold for 1 second. Slowly lower your arm down to your side (start position).

▌ Now raise and supinate your left arm. Lower.

▌ This completes 1 repetition.

▌ Repeat until fatigued.

▌ Perform 2 sets.

LATERAL ARM RAISE

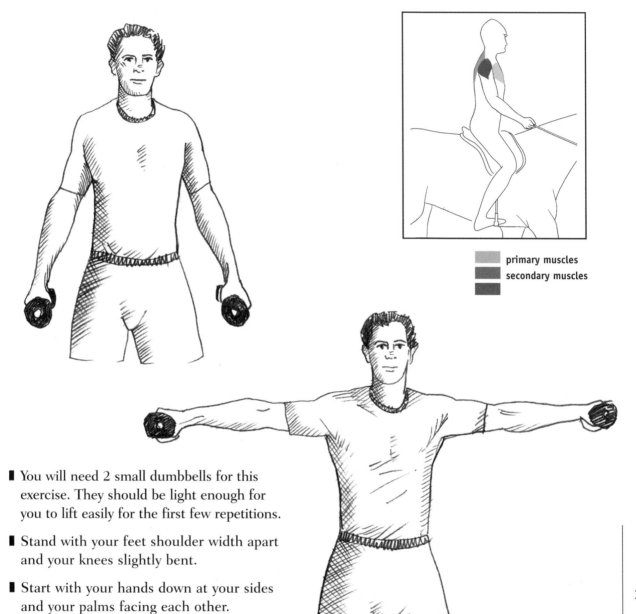

■ primary muscles
■ secondary muscles
■

- You will need 2 small dumbbells for this exercise. They should be light enough for you to lift easily for the first few repetitions.

- Stand with your feet shoulder width apart and your knees slightly bent.

- Start with your hands down at your sides and your palms facing each other.

- Breathing normally, slowly raise your arms until they are parallel to the floor. Keep your shoulders down and back.

- Hold for 1 second. Slowly lower your arms down to your side (start position).

- This completes 1 repetition.

- Repeat until fatigue.

- Perform 2 sets.

37

KICK-BACKS

Y OUR TRICEPS' FUNCTION is to extend your arms at your elbows. The Kick-backs will improve the strength and muscular endurance in your triceps and will help you maintain correct muscle balance with your biceps.

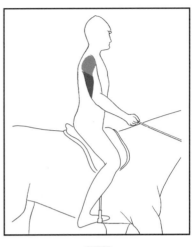

primary muscles

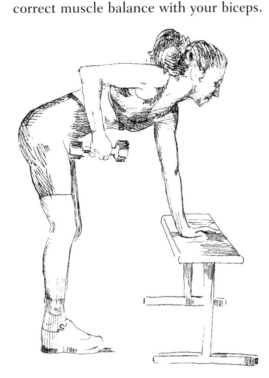

▌ Bend over and lean against a chair or bench with your left hand. Your back should be parallel to the floor and your knees bent. Grasp the dumbbell in your right hand and bend your elbow until your right upper arm is parallel to the floor and your elbow is tucked close to your side. This is your start position.

▌ Keeping your upper arm motionless, slowly straighten your arm to full extension. Focus on and squeeze your triceps especially at the top of your motion.

▌ Hold for 1 second, then return to the start position.

▌ Repeat until fatigued.

▌ Repeat with your left arm for an equal number of repetitions to complete 1 set.

▌ Perform 2 sets.

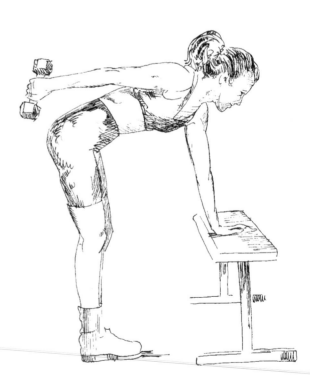

OVERHEAD EXTENSIONS

ALTERNATE

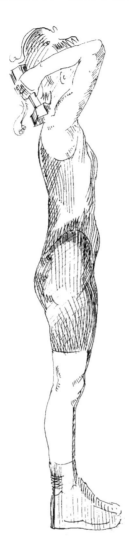
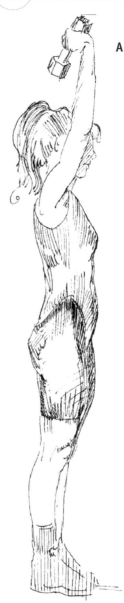

▌ Stand or sit on a bench with your back straight and your feet flat on the floor.

▌ Holding the dumbbell in your right hand, raise your right arm straight above your head.

▌ Support your right arm with your left hand by grasping your right upper arm just below the elbow.

▌ Slowly bend your right arm at the elbow until your forearm is parallel to the floor.

▌ Return to full extension.

▌ This completes 1 repetition.

▌ Breathe normally and squeeze your triceps throughout each repetition.

▌ Repeat until fatigue.

▌ Repeat with your left arm for an equal number of repetitions to complete 1 set.

▌ Perform 2 sets.

ROTATION CURL

YOUR BICEPS AND YOUR BRACHIALIS flex your arms at your elbows and assist in shoulder flexion (raising your arm) and in shoulder adduction (moving your arm across your body). The Biceps Rotation Curl adds strength and muscular endurance from 2 separate angles, working both your biceps and your brachialis muscles.

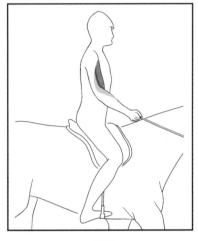

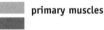
primary muscles

- Stand with your feet shoulder width-apart and your knees slightly bent.

- Hold a dumbbell in each hand and let your arms hang at your sides with your palms facing each other.

- Flexing at the elbow, raise the right dumbbell toward your shoulder.

- Keep your elbow as stationary as possible and exhale as you curl.

- Rotate your palm up toward the sky as you near the halfway point of your curl.

- Squeeze your biceps throughout the entire curl.

- When you reach the top, squeeze for 1 second then slowly lower your dumbbell.

- Repeat with your left arm to complete 1 repetition.

- Repeat until fatigued.

HAMMER CURL

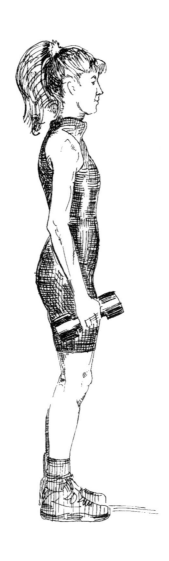
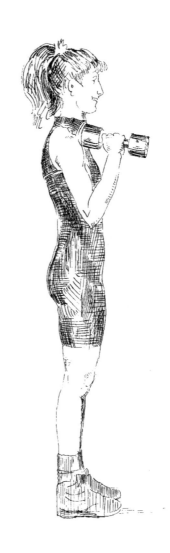

▌ Stand with your feet shoulder width-apart and your knees slightly bent.

▌ Hold a dumbbell in each hand and let your arms hang at your sides. As in the Rotation Curl, your palms should face each other.

▌ Flexing at the elbow, raise the right dumbbell toward your shoulder.

▌ Keep your elbow as stationary as possible and exhale as you curl.

▌ Keep your thumb toward the sky and your palm facing inside as you curl.

▌ Squeeze your biceps throughout the entire curl.

▌ When you reach the top squeeze for 1 second then slowly lower your dumbbell.

▌ Repeat with your left arm to complete 1 repetition.

▌ Repeat until fatigued. Perform 2 sets.

WRIST SWING

UNIVERSAL

T HE WRIST SWING IS THE FIRST of the Good Hands exercises. It is designed to help you develop softer and more precise hands in the saddle by building strength and muscular endurance in the brachioradialis muscles in your forearms, by reinforcing correct hand-wrist-arm positioning (enabling you to avoid rolling your hands over), and by improving your muscle awareness.

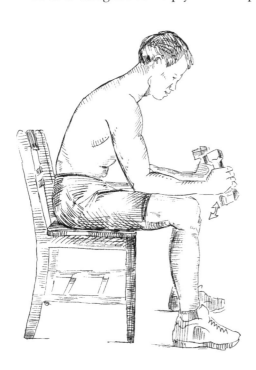

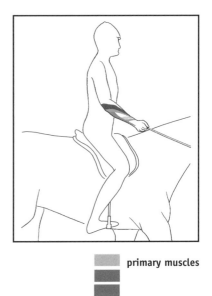

primary muscles

- You will need a hammer (or light-weight dumbbells) and a bench for this exercise.

- Sit on the bench and rest your forearms on your thighs.

- Holding the hammer in your left hand with your palms facing each other, slowly swing your left wrist up and down until you reach fatigue.

- Repeat exercise with your right hand.

   Try these variations:

- Hold dumbbells in both hands with your palms facing the floor. Slowly swing your weights up and down until you again reach fatigue. (Repeating the exercise with your palms down works your wrist extensors for muscle balance.) Your movements should be smooth and controlled.

- Perform a total of 2 sets.

42

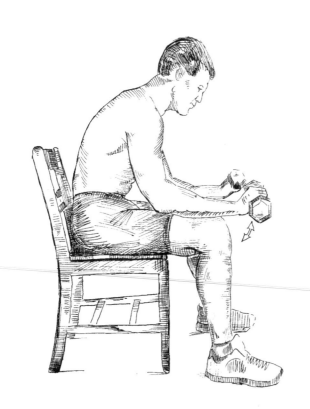

ORANGE CRUSH

HEAVY HANDS COMBINED WITH a negative attitude in the saddle only serves to injure and toughen your horse's mouth. However, adequate strength in your hands and forearms can enhance the development and effective use of soft-precise hands in the saddle. The Orange Crush will add strength and muscular endurance to your forearms, and improve the strength, muscular awareness, and dexterity in your hands. Combine good hands with a positive and patient mental approach and eventually you and your horse will have fewer differences-of-opinion.

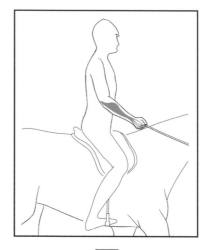

primary muscles

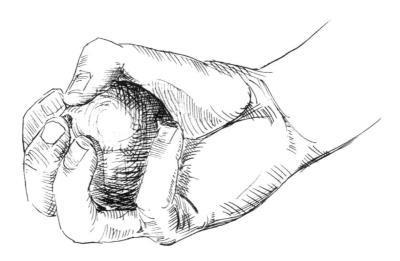

43

▌ Grasp a tennis ball in your right hand.

▌ Squeeze and hold for 1 second, then release.

▌ Repeat until fatigue.

▌ Perform an equal number of repetitions with your left hand to complete 1 set.

▌ Perform a total of 2 sets.

STEEPLE

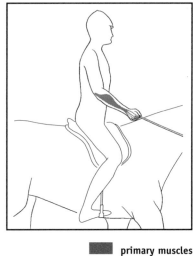

primary muscles

THE PROBLEM WITH HOLDING a pair of reins is that the movement in your fingers must be very subtle or control of the reins shifts from your hands-wrists to your shoulders-upper arms. The result: You overreact in your cues. The Steeple is derived from a traditional children's game. It works to develop dexterity and muscular awareness in your fingers. This will improve the precision in your hand movements helping you become more accurate in your cues and more responsive to your horse's mouth.

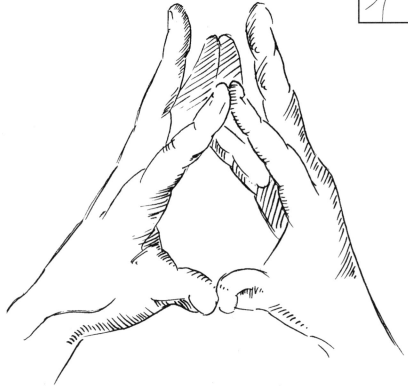

- Hold your hands together and align the corresponding fingers.

- Separate your palms with your fingers still touching.

- Lift your thumbs apart and hold for 1 second, then touch them together again.

- Lift your index fingers apart and hold for 1 second, then return ... lift your middle (3rd) fingers apart, hold, return ... lift your ring (4th) fingers apart ... lift your little (5th) fingers apart ....

- Repeat for 1 minute.

- This completes 1 set.

44

REIN WALK

You will need a pair of reins for this exercise.

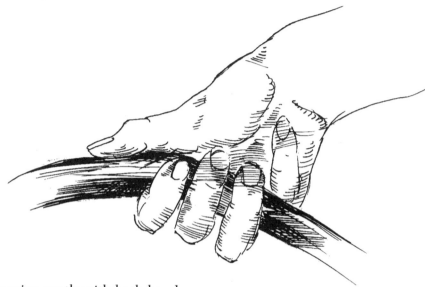

▌ Grasp the reins gently with both hands, placing your thumbs and little fingers on the top of the reins and your other fingers on the bottom side.

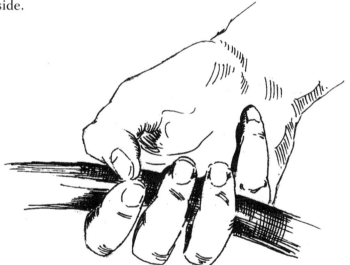

▌ Now bend your thumbs and slide your fingers and slowly "walk" the reins through your fingers.

▌ Continue exercise for at least 1 minute.

▌ Perform a total of 2 sets.

45

SEAT-SPECIFIC EXERCISES

SEVERAL OF THE RIDING STYLES targeted in this book present physical challenges unique to that particular seat. To meet these demands, The Equestrian Workout offers three seat-specific exercises on pages 47–49 designed to help you enhance the physical qualities unique to your specific style of riding.

Targeted riding styles include:

▌ Forward seat (hunter, jumper, english pleasure, etc.)

▌ Balanced seat (dressage, western, gymkhana, etc.)

▌ Saddleseat

Choose the one exercise that applies to your style of riding. This will conclude your strength and muscular endurance exercises. Follow immediately with the flexibility-posture and balance exercises.

EXTREME SKIER

FORWARD SEAT RIDERS commonly sway their backs when riding over fences and during posting. Unfortunately, holding this position quickly fatigues the muscles in your lower back which is a primary reason why the most common complaint among forward seat riders is lower back soreness. The Extreme Skier further addresses this problem by providing additional exercise to build critical muscle endurance in your lower back and hips. Secondary emphasis is in your quadriceps muscles.

Note: Strong abdominal muscles share the load of holding your back and pelvis in correct position, so work hard on your abdominal exercises.

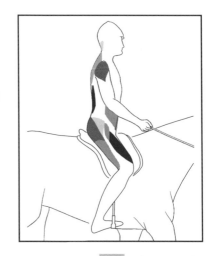

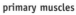 primary muscles

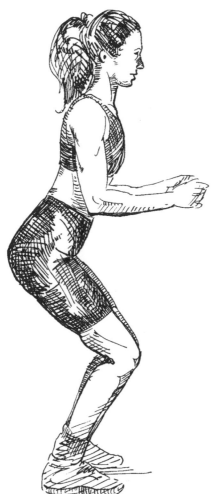

- Stand with your feet shoulder-width apart and your knees bent to a 45-degree angle.

- Position your hands in front of your body as if you were holding a pair or reins.

- Push your butt out behind you and sway your back. Breathe normally and focus on the muscles in your lower back.

- Hold this position for a minimum of 1 minute.

47

ABDUCTOR LIFT

As a BALANCED SEAT RIDER, you are occasionally faced with opening your upper legs while maintaining sufficient lower leg contact to encourage your horse to relax and move forward at the same time. This can be a physically difficult cue to perform. While you do not need to be a contortionist to pull this off, you do require sufficient flexibility throughout your body and adequate strength in your outer thigh muscles (abductors). The Abductor Lift works to build strength and muscular endurance in your abductors.

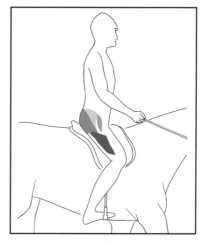

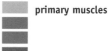
primary muscles

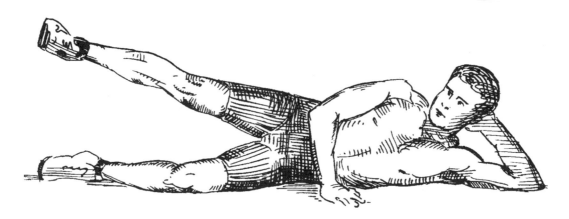

- Lie down on your left side with your right (upper) leg fully extended.
- Your left (lower) leg should be bent at the knee and your hips should be in a vertical line.
- Slowly lift your right (upper) leg as high as is comfortable.
- Hold for 1 second then lower to complete 1 repetition.
- Breathe normally and squeeze your abductor muscle as you exercise.
- Repeat until you reach fatigue.
- Roll over and repeat exercise with your left leg for an equal number of repetitions.
- Perform 2 sets.

FLARED LEG LIFT

ADDLESEAT RIDERS MUST RIDE with a unique leg position opposite to other styles of riding: The inside edges of your feet are flared out. This requires considerable flexibility along the inside of your ankle and increased strength along the outside of your ankle. The Adductor Stretch and Ham Stretch are also particularly beneficial for saddleseat riders.

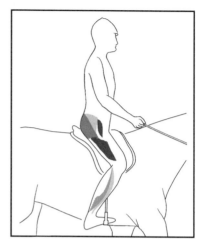

primary muscles

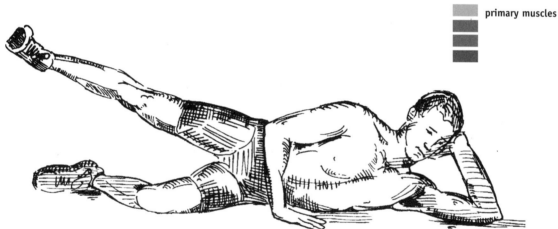

▌ Lie down on your left side with your legs extended. Your hips should be in a vertical line.

▌ Lift your right (upper) leg a comfortable distance off of the floor.

▌ Point the inside edge of your foot and your heel as you lift your leg.

▌ Hold for 1 second, then lower.

▌ Repeat until fatigue.

▌ Repeat exercise with your left leg for an equal number of repetitions.

Note: Here is an excellent exercise you can perform in addition to the Flared Leg Lift.

You will need a bicycle tube or surgical tubing tied in a loop. Sit in a chair and place your foot in the tubing. Pull to increase the tension. Start with your foot turned in then slowly turn your foot out as far as is comfortable. Repeat until you reach fatigue then perform the exercise with your other foot.

49

FLEXIBILITY & POSTURE EXERCISES

IMPROVED FLEXIBILITY is the cornerstone of your success as a rider-athlete:

▌ It reduces the potential for injuries. Increased flexibility enables your body joints to withstand greater impact-shock when your body encounters an unyielding surface ... such as the ground.

▌ It contributes to improved athletic performance. The rider-athlete with good flexibility has greater freedom of movement in all directions, and can more easily change the direction of a movement, decreasing the chance of a fall, and the chance of injury when a fall occurs.

The New Equestrian Workout emphasizes a highly effective and safe form of "static stretching." This is stretching your muscle to the point of mild discomfort and holding that position for at least 45 seconds.

▌ The minimum stretching time of 45 seconds is emphasized because when you attempt to stretch, sensory impulses from your central nervous system cause your muscle to contract and resist the stretch for 30 seconds. Only after you have held the stretch continuously for 30 seconds are new sensory messages released causing that muscle to finally relax and lengthen.

Here are some guidelines to successful stretching:

▌ Gently hold your stretch. Never bounce.

▌ Begin with an easy stretch, then proceed to moderate stretches.

▌ Avoid severe stretching. You should experience only mild discomfort during stretching, never sharp pain.

▌ Breathe in a relaxed and rhythmic manner. Never hold your breath.

▌ Stretch every day. Studies show that daily stretching will produce significant improvement in flexibility.

▌ Stretching is excellent for injury prevention only when combined with strength exercises.

You will conclude with the balance exercises on pages 69–74. The first and foremost comment on balance is simply: You can never have enough!

Helpful balancing hints:

▌ Always look straight ahead, never down at your feet.

▌ Keep your knees bent slightly.

▌ If you are having trouble balancing, don't get frustrated. Slow down, relax, breathe deeply, and keep trying. Eventually you will succeed!

▌ All of the balancing exercises are great for injury prevention, but if you already have a serious injury, consult with a professional before attempting any balance exercises.

DORSAL FLEX

THE AVERAGE AMERICAN and by extension the average rider is woefully weak and inflexible in his/her lower back muscles. So, it's not surprising that the most common complaint among competitive equestrians is chronic pain in the lower back. Maintaining correct riding posture strains your lower back muscles to the point of fatigue, and every stride of your horse transmits tiny shock waves through your lower back and up your spine. So how do you avoid chronic lower back pain? The answer is: Increase your abdominal and back strength, muscular endurance, and flexibility.

The Dorsal Flex is designed to stretch your lower back muscles and hip flexors with a secondary emphasis in your hamstrings and quadriceps. Increased flexibility will reduce fatigue and soreness in your lower back and will help you develop a deeper riding seat.

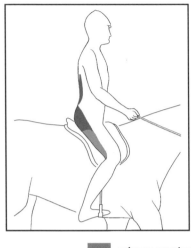

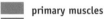 primary muscles

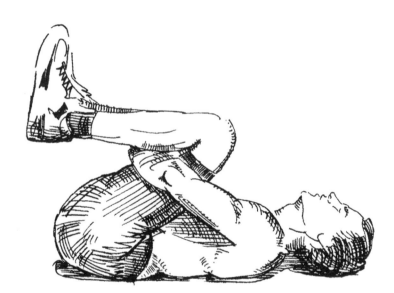

▌ Lie flat on your back with your legs extended. Your breathing should be relaxed and rhythmic.

▌ Slowly bring both knees to your chest, clasping the back of your thighs with your hands.

▌ Focus on the stretch in your lower back muscles as you gently pull your knees further into your chest.

▌ Hold this position for a minimum of 45 seconds.

51

CROSS-LEGGED BOW

INTERMEDIATE–ADVANCED

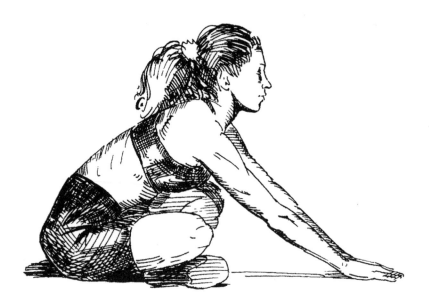

■ Sit cross-legged on the floor.

■ Sit as tall as you can up on your seat bones ... this will help you maintain correct posture.

■ With your hands on your knees, slowly bend forward at the hips ... keep your back straight as you flex gently forward.

■ Hold for a minimum of 45 seconds.

■ After stretching in position 1 for 45 seconds, lower your head, relax, and let your back round up toward the sky.

■ Extend your arms forward and gently reach toward the floor.

■ Hold this position for another 30 seconds.

Try these variations:

1. Slowly let your head drop to the floor. Hold.

2. Rotate your torso so that your hands extend past your left knee, Repeat to your right. Hold.

VENTRAL STRETCH

BEGINNER

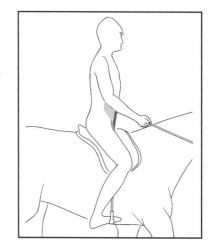

THE PREVIOUS EXERCISES, The Dorsal Flex and The Cross-legged Bow, stretch your back dorsally. The Ventral Stretch is designed to stretch your lower back in a "ventral" or frontal direction. Why stretch both ways? Because your back needs to be equally flexible in both directions to allow you to move freely through a full range of motion and to comfortably maintain correct posture.

Here's a fact to remember: Most back problems are at least partially caused by dorsal/ventral inflexibility. Consequently, this exercise focuses heavily on properly stretching and conditioning your back so that you may spend quality time in the saddle for many years to come.

 primary muscles

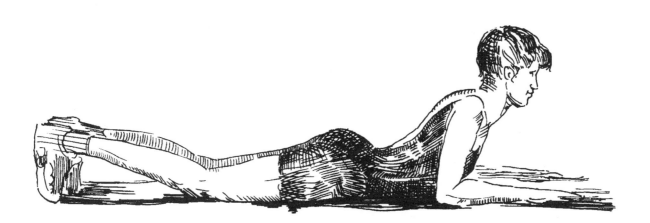

- Lie face down on the floor.

- Place your hands shoulder width apart and parallel with your face.

- Keeping your hips firmly on the floor, gently sway your back and raise up onto your elbows and forearms.

- Breathe in a slow and rhythmic manner to help yourself relax and remember to concentrate on your back muscles as you stretch.

- Hold this position for at least 45 seconds.

53

VENTRAL STRETCH

INTERMEDIATE–ADVANCED

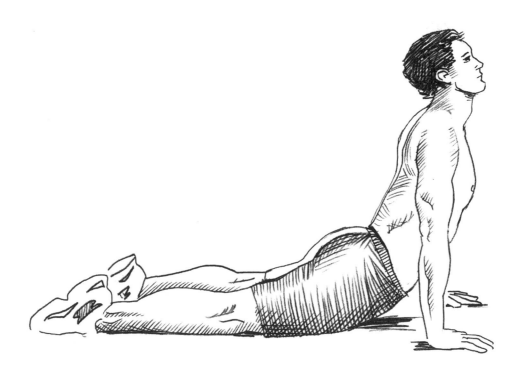

- Assume the same position shown in the beginner Ventral Stretch. Shift your weight off your elbows and onto your hands and slowly raise your elbows off of the floor for a deeper stretch.

- The more you straighten your arms, the more of a stretch you will experience.

- Remember to keep your hips on the floor, focus, and breathe in a relaxed, rhythmic manner.

ANGRY CAT & SWAY-BACK HORSE

UNIVERSAL

POOR POSTURE is a common equestrian condition. Riders often collapse their chests and round their shoulders forward instead of sitting "tall" in the saddle. Contributing causes to poor posture are a lack of muscle awareness, inflexibility across the chest, weak back muscles, and inflexibility though the entire back. All of these areas will be addressed in this workout, but we'll concentrate on back inflexibility for one more exercise. One of the best methods for increasing your overall back flexibility is a traditional children's exercise called the Angry Cat & Sway-back Horse. This exercise will stretch muscles dorsally the entire length of your back, and ventrally through your abdomen. As you perform this exercise you'll quickly understand how it earned its name.

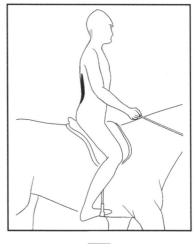

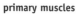 primary muscles

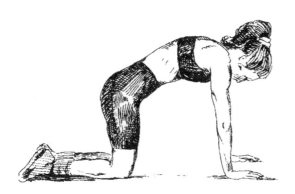

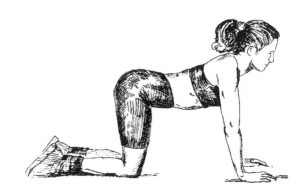

- Lower yourself onto all fours, placing your hands and your knees shoulder width apart.

- Slowly arch your back toward the sky until you have reached as far as you can go. Face the floor to minimize stress on your neck. This is the "Angry Cat" position. (Note: Spitting and clawing are not required for authenticity's sake, although they may prove to be effective stress relievers and/or self-defense mechanisms.)

- Hold this position for a minimum of 45 seconds, then proceed directly to step 2.

- Starting from the Angry-Cat position, gently sway your back down towards the floor until you have comfortably reached the limit of your range of motion.

- Face slightly forward to minimize stress on your neck. This is the "Sway-back Horse."

- Breathe normally and hold this position for a minimum of 45 seconds.

55

REACH-FOR-THE-SKY

A<small>T FIRST GLANCE</small> this posture exercise appears to be extremely easy. But it may surprise you, it's tougher than it looks. Reach-for-the-Sky is designed to increase the flexibility primarily in your upper back with secondary emphasis in your chest. So, you're wondering how flexibility affects your posture? Stretching effectively extends your range of motion which enables you to maintain good posture more comfortably. As a result, you will maintain better posture more consistently. (Similar to a domino effect.) Reach-for-the-Sky also serves as an excellent test to occasionally gauge your posture level.

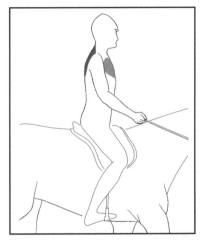

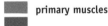
primary muscles

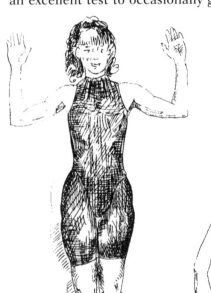

▮ Stand with your back against a flat wall with your elbows pointing out to the sides and your hands pointing up. Now here begins the tough part.

▮ Touch the wall on 5 points:

  1. the heels of your feet

  2. your buttocks

  3. your shoulders

  4. your elbows

  5. the top of your hands

▮ If you can't touch on all 5 points, get as close as you can and proceed with the exercise. Attempt to keep your back straight throughout the entire exercise.

▮ Slowly slide your hands up as high as you can reach and lightly touch your index fingers together.

▮ Breathe normally and hold this position for a minimum of 45 seconds.

  Note: Any resemblance to the position assumed by victims of the medieval torture device known as "the rack" is purely coincidental.

HIP STRETCH

Y OUR HIP EXTENSORS ALLOW YOU to extend your legs at your hips, enabling you to perform necessary functions such as walking and mounting your horse. The Hip Stretch is designed to stretch your hip extensors with secondary emphasis in your gluteus medius. Improved flexibility in your hip extensors will help you develop a deeper seat for riding.

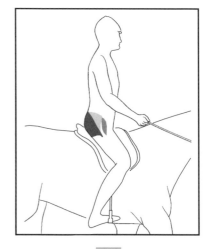

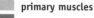 primary muscles

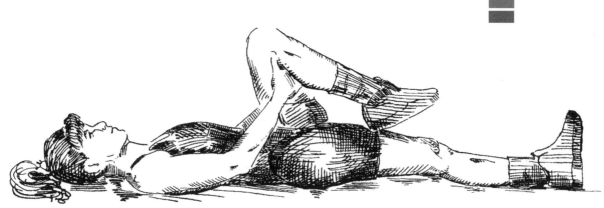

- Lie flat on your back with your legs extended.

- Keep your head flat on the floor.

- Clasp the back of your left thigh with both hands and slowly bring your knee towards your chest as far as it will comfortably travel.

- Hold for a minimum of 45 seconds.

- Breathe normally and try to visualize your hip flexors and lower back muscles relax-

ing and lengthening as you gently hold your stretch. Remember, never rock back and forth during a stretch, all stretching should be slow and controlled.

- Gently return your left leg to the extended position.

- Repeat the stretch with your right leg.

57

RUNNER'S STRETCH

Your hip flexors are the antagonistic muscles to your hip extensors and perform the opposite action. Your hip flexors enable you to flex your leg at the hip, which allows you to walk, run, and lift your leg into a stirrup. The Runner's Stretch stretches your hip flexors with secondary emphasis in your groin and hamstrings. As with your hip extensors, improved flexibility in your hip flexors will help you develop a deeper seat for riding. This exercise will also help prevent lower back pain.

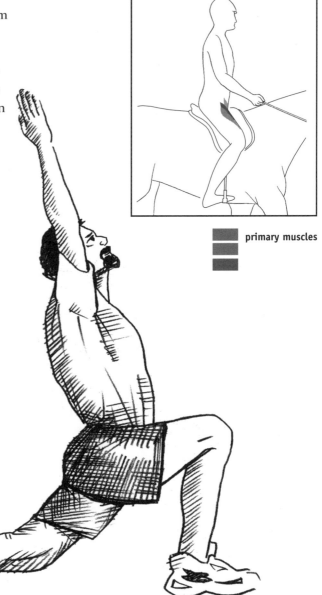

primary muscles

■ Start on hands and knees, then place your left foot flat on the floor directly under your left knee. Slide your right foot back extending your right leg behind you as far as possible.

■ Keep your upper body upright and place your hands on your left knee.

■ Allow your hips to sink down and forward toward your left heel.

■ Hold this position for at least 45 seconds.

■ Repeat with your right foot forward.

■ To improve your balance, perform exercise with your hands extended over your head and your palms facing each other.

SEATED HAM STRETCH

Y OUR HAMSTRING ACTS AS a large biceps between your knee and hip and enables you to flex your leg at the knee. It plays a crucial role in daily activities such as walking and running. While it is not one of the primary muscles used during riding, it is employed whenever you attempt to lengthen your leg and lower your heel in the stirrup. In addition, it is necessary to stretch and strengthen your hamstrings to maintain adequate leg muscle balance and overall fitness.

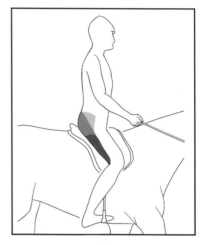

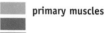 primary muscles

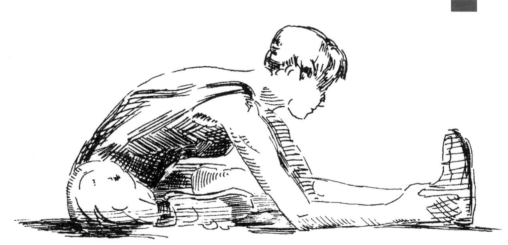

59

- Sit down on the floor with both legs stretched in front of you.

- Slide your right foot up your left leg until it rests next to your left knee. Keeping your back straight and bending only at the hips, slowly reach for your left ankle with both hands. Try to feel your left hamstring relaxing and lengthening as you stretch. Remember, stretch only until you feel mild discomfort (never pain!) in your hamstring, and don't bounce!

- Hold this position for a minimum of 45 seconds.

- Relax and repeat with your right hamstring.

STANDING HAM STRETCH

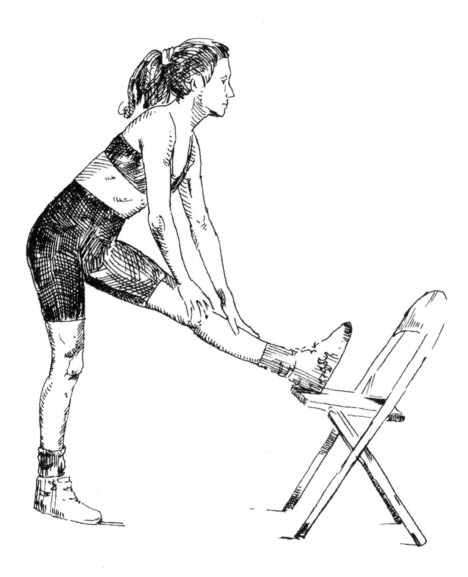

▌ For this exercise you will need to use an object that is knee to hip high such as a chair, table, or even 2 stacked hay bales.

▌ Place your left foot on top of the object, keeping your left leg as straight as you can. It is okay to bend slightly at the knees if you must.

▌ Slowly bend forward at the hip (keep your back straight), look straight ahead, and

reach for your ankles with both hands. All motion should be smooth and controlled.

▌ Hold for a minimum of 45 seconds, then stretch your right hamstring.

QUAD STRETCH

UNIVERSAL

YOUR QUADRICEPS IS THE ANTAGONISTIC MUSCLE to your hamstring, performing the opposite action of extending your leg at the knee. You use your quadriceps during riding whenever you post a trot or "lengthen" your leg in the saddle.

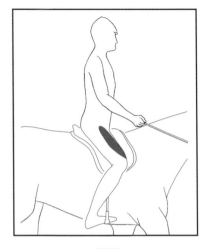

primary muscles

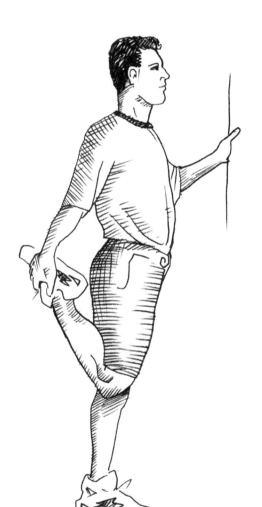

▌ Stand next to a wall or post and use your right hand to maintain your balance.

▌ Bend your right knee and grasp your right ankle with your left hand.

▌ Slowly pull your heel up and toward your buttocks until you feel a stretch in your quadriceps muscle. Keep your knees together.

▌ Hold this position for a minimum of 45 seconds.

▌ Lower and repeat with your left leg.

SUMO STRETCH

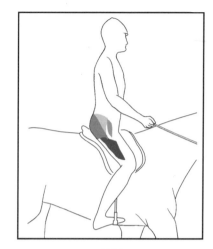

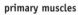
primary muscles

Y OUR "ADDUCTORS" OR INNER THIGH MUSCLES help you maintain your balance when standing, walking, or running, a role that goes largely unnoticed and doesn't require a great deal of endurance or strength. Consequently, most individuals' adductors are weak and under-developed. During riding, your adductors play a starring role requiring a great amount of endurance and strength. Flexibility is needed to reduce the amount of stress and fatigue your adductors incur when applying some of that strength during leg-cueing, collection, riding in a forward seat, or when you're just hanging on for the ride.

Note: For those of you with visions of traditional wrestling fame, this is an opportune moment to stamp your feet and growl something menacing in Japanese.

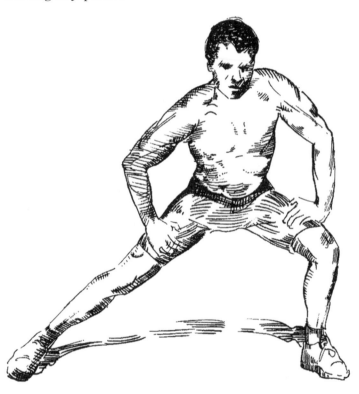

▪ Stand with your feet spread wide apart and place your hands above your knees.

▪ Keeping both soles of your feet planted firmly on the floor, gently shift your weight onto your right leg, bend your right knee and straighten your left knee. (Do not bend your left knee past 90 degrees as this will place additional and unnecessary stress on your knee joint.)

▪ Breathe normally and attempt to feel your adductor muscle as it lengthens.

▪ Hold steadily for a minimum of 45 seconds, then repeat with your right leg extended.

ADDUCTOR STRETCH

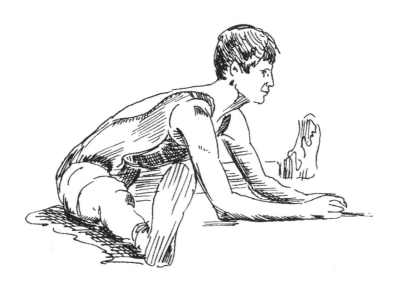

- Sit on the floor and spread your legs apart.

- Your knees should be straight.

- Slowly bend forward at the hips, keeping your back straight and your head up.

- Breathe in a relaxed and rhythmic manner and focus on your adductor muscles as they begin to lengthen. As with many other body parts, your adductor muscles can become strained rather easily so be smart and stretch gently and patiently.

- Hold this position for a minimum of 45 seconds.

PUSH-THE-WALL-DOWN

ANYONE WHO HAS TAKEN riding lessons knows well the incessant bark of the instructor commanding them to lower their heels. The inability to maintain a proper heel angle is a result of inflexible calf muscles. Push-the-Wall-Down will improve your flexibility in your gastrocnemius muscles which are the most recognizable part of your calves.

The combination of this exercise and the Soleus Stretch (next page) will enable you to develop a greater range of motion and help you maintain a correct riding form which may satisfy even your riding instructor.

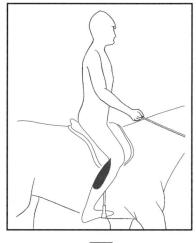

primary muscles

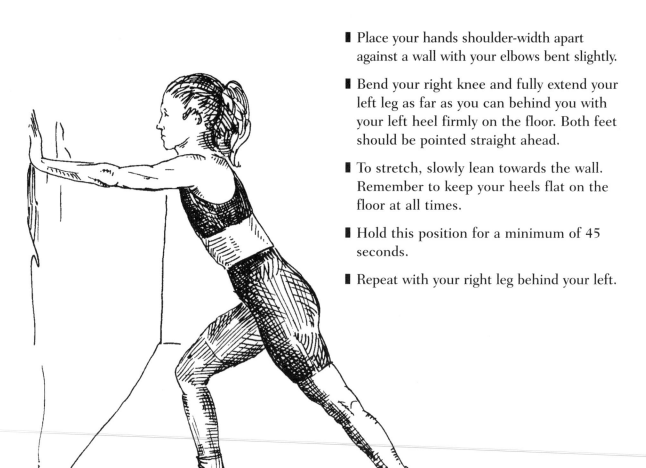

▌ Place your hands shoulder-width apart against a wall with your elbows bent slightly.

▌ Bend your right knee and fully extend your left leg as far as you can behind you with your left heel firmly on the floor. Both feet should be pointed straight ahead.

▌ To stretch, slowly lean towards the wall. Remember to keep your heels flat on the floor at all times.

▌ Hold this position for a minimum of 45 seconds.

▌ Repeat with your right leg behind your left.

SOLEUS STRETCH

UNIVERSAL

THE SOLEUS STRETCH IS DESIGNED to increase your flexibility in your other calf muscle, the lesser known but highly important soleus.

Successful track and field athletes have learned that the most effective method of improving calf flexibility is to separately stretch the gastrocnemius and soleus muscles. Equestrians athletes can benefit greatly from this knowledge as well.

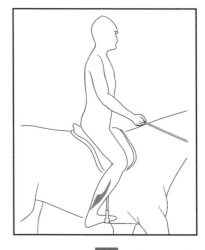

primary muscles

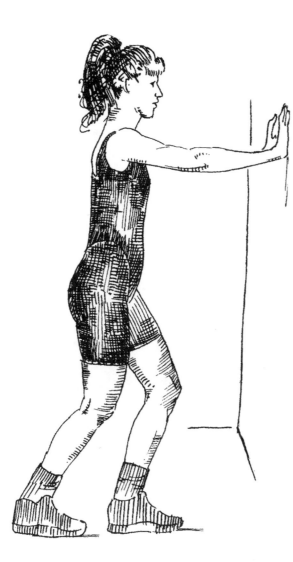

▌ Place your hands shoulder-width apart against a wall. Your elbows should be slightly bent.

▌ Position your right foot comfortably behind your left foot with your right heel firmly on the floor. Both feet should be pointed straight ahead.

▌ Bend slowly at your knees, stopping as soon as your right heel begins to lift off of the floor. Do not permit your heel to actually rise, it is important to keep it flat on the floor to gain full benefit of this exercise. All of your movements should be smooth and controlled.

▌ Breathe normally and hold this position for a minimum of 45 seconds.

▌ Repeat with your left leg behind your right.

65

CHEST   *The New Total Rider*

DOORWAY STRETCH

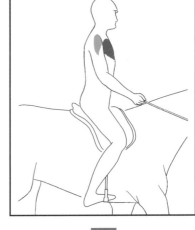

THE DOORWAY STRETCH IS DESIGNED to improve your posture by increasing the flexibility in your pectorals (chest) and anterior deltoids (front shoulder). When combined with strengthening exercises for your upper back this exercise will help you break the habit of rolling your shoulders forward and collapsing your chest when you ride.

Note: definition of the trainer's seat = legs overbent, body slanted forward, elbows pointed out, shoulders rounded, chest collapsed, and eyes down. Quote this to your trainer at your own peril!

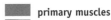 primary muscles

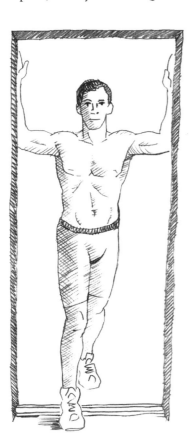

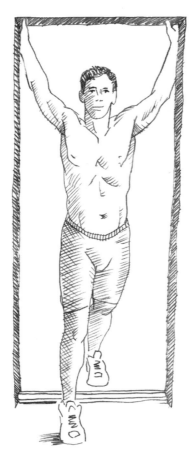

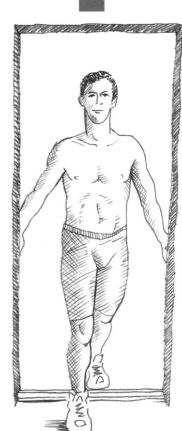

▮ Stand inside a doorway with one foot through the doorway and one foot behind.

▮ Place your hands on each side of the doorway at shoulder height with your elbows at 90 degrees.

▮ Gently lean forward. You should feel compression between your shoulder blades and slight stretching across your chest.

▮ Hold this position for a minimum of 45 seconds.

▮ Try sliding your hands to the top corners of the doorway.

▮ Place your hands on the doorway by your hips.

7TH-INNING STRETCH

UNIVERSAL

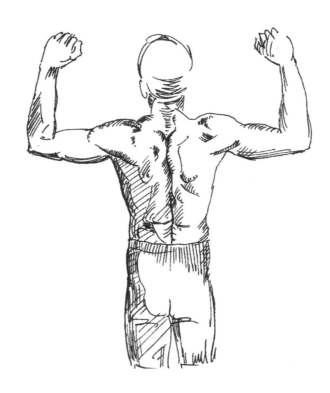

- Maintaining good posture, stand or sit on a chair or the floor.

- Raise your arms out to your sides.

- Bend your elbows 90 degrees with your fingers pointing up and your upper arms parallel to the floor.

- Simultaneously bring both arms back and squeeze your shoulder blades together. You should also feel a slight stretch across your chest.

- Hold this position for at least 45 seconds.

REALLY-OLD RELAXATION TECHNIQUE

THIS SIMPLE BUT EFFECTIVE breathing exercise has its roots in ancient arts such as Yoga, Tai Chi, and Aikido. You will use it as part of this workout to prepare yourself for balancing. Proper breath control enhances your ability to balance by helping your body and mind relax. This will enable you to focus (and balance) more effectively:

- Stand with your feet shoulder-width apart and your knees unlocked. Let your arms hang at your sides and focus your eyes forward.

- Slowly inhale as deeply as you can. Allow your shoulders to gently rise with each intake of breath.

- Exhale slowly and let your shoulders drop softly as a feather. Imagine your physical and mental stress being carried out on each expulsion of breath. Feel the tension drain from your body and from your mind.

- Repeat at least 3 times.

  Note: Use this relaxation technique anytime you feel tense.

THE STORK

A HIGHLY DEVELOPED SENSE OF BALANCE is among the most important qualities possessed by the average person and the successful rider. Without it you would be unable to sit, stand, or walk, much less ride a horse. The ability to balance is created from a combination of muscle awareness, muscle conditioning, and electrical signals to/from your central nervous system. Effective balance is not a given trait, it is learned and developed. Inactivity breeds poor balance. On the other hand, focused training produces excellent balancing ability.

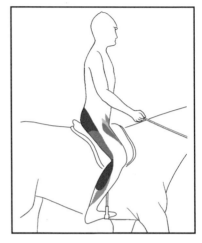

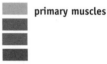

primary muscles

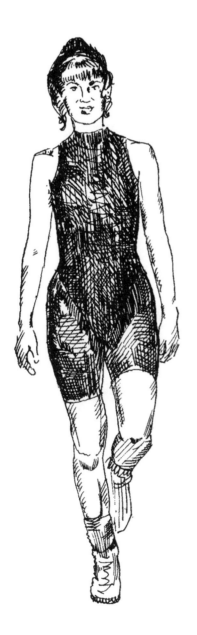

Prepare for balancing by performing the Really-Old Relaxation Technique on page 68.

- Stand with your feet shoulder-width apart and your knees unlocked.

- Face forward and let your arms hang at your sides.

- Shift your weight to your left leg and slowly raise your right foot off of the floor. It's hard, but try to avoid the temptation to look down at your feet, and do not allow your legs to touch each other.*

- Breathe normally and attempt to balance for a minimum of 1 minute.

- Repeat, raising your left foot.

69

THE STORK

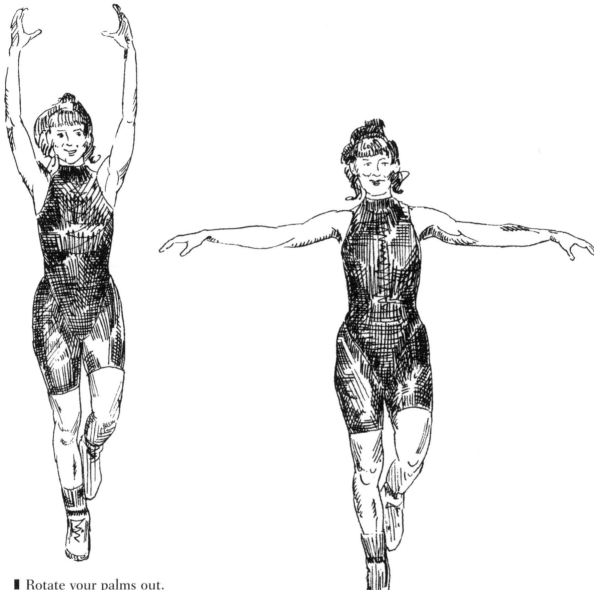

70

- ▌ Rotate your palms out.

- ▌ Exhaling softly, gently lower your arms back to your sides.

- ▌ Repeat 6 times without lowering your raised foot to the floor.

- ▌ Repeat the entire exercise with your left foot raised.

For an **Advanced-Level** balancing exercise, perform the beginner Stork (on page 67) with your eyes closed. Sound easy? You may be surprised.

THE 10-TOE CONSPIRACY

When your legs touch they communicate, conspire, and assist each other in responding to the demands encountered during an activity such as balancing. (Similar to cheating during your biology exam.) This makes a balancing exercise easier, but less efficient in improving your skills.

STANDING BALANCE BOARD

BEGINNER

THE STANDING BALANCE BOARD offers a challenging alternative to The Stork. As the name implies, it requires an easily-constructed prop called a balance board. For instructions on how to construct a balance board, see Building A Balance Board on page 127.

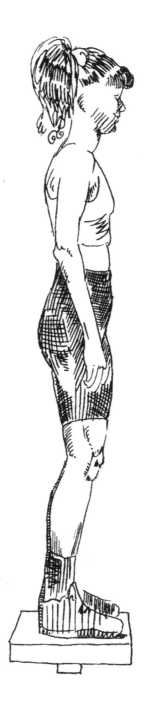

Prepare for balancing by performing the Really-Old Relaxation Technique on page 68.

▮ Place the balance board on the floor with the beam running left-right.

▮ Center your feet on the board. Your feet should be approximately shoulder-width apart, and your knees should be unlocked.

▮ Let your arms hang lazily at your sides.

▮ Focus your eyes straight ahead. (Pretend you are standing on the high-dive at the swimming pool for the first time: Don't look down!)

▮ Breathe normally, and remember … by relaxing your body and your mind you will enhance your ability to balance.

▮ Attempt to balance for for a minimum of 1 minute.

▮ Repeat the exercise with the balance board running front-back.

Feeling frustrated with your attempts to balance? Simply take 2–3 long, deep breaths, exhale slowly, R-E-L-A-X, and try again. Eventually you will succeed.

71

STANDING BALANCE BOARD INTERMEDIATE–ADVANCED

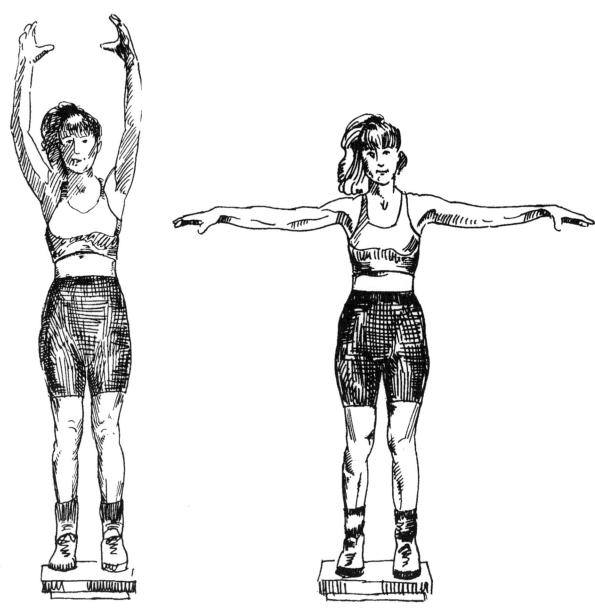

▌ Center yourself on the board as detailed in the beginner Standing Balance Board on the previous page.

▌ Turn your palms outward and inhale gently as you raise both arms slowly from your sides until your palms touch high above your head.

▌ Rotate your palms out. Exhaling softly, lower your arms gently to your sides. Repeat.

▌ Attempt to balance for a minimum of 1 minute while performing steps 1 & 2.

For an **Advanced-Level** balancing exercise, perform the beginner Standing Balance Board with your eyes closed.

KNEELING BALANCE BOARD

THE KNEELING BALANCE BOARD offers a sport-specific balancing exercise by lowering your center of gravity and encouraging you to utilize your upper legs and seat for balance. This exercise requires the use of a balance board (see Building A Balance Board, p. 119) and a small, soft pillow.

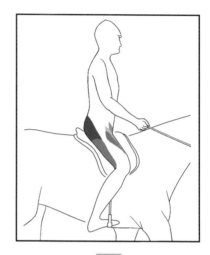

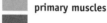 primary muscles

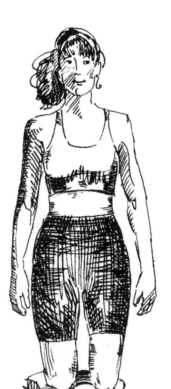

- Using the pillow as a cushion, kneel on the balance board with the center beam running front to back between your knees.

- Space your knees shoulder width apart.

- With your arms at your sides, raise your feet off of the floor and attempt to balance on your knees for a minimum of 1 minute.

- Focus your eyes straight ahead and breathe normally.

- As you become more adept at balancing, attempt to balance longer—up to 3 minutes.

CAUTION

Discontinue immediately if you experience any knee pain or have a history of knee problems.

73

KNEELING BALANCE BOARD   INTERMEDIATE–ADVANCED

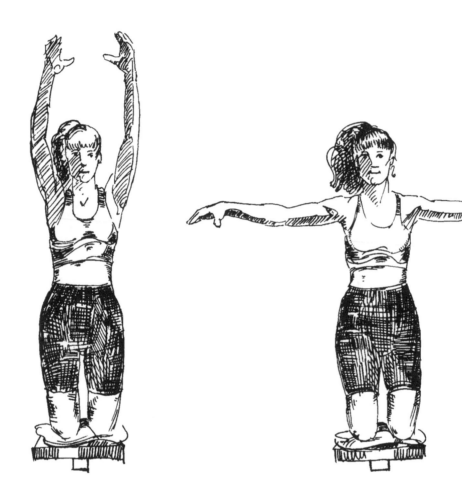

■ Center yourself on the board as detailed in the beginner Kneeling Balance Board on the previous page.

■ Turn your palms outward and inhale gently as you raise both arms slowly until your palms touch high above your head.

■ Rotate your palms out.

■ Exhaling softly, gently lower your arms until your fingertips touch the floor.

■ Repeat.

■ Attempt to balance for a minimum of 1 minute while performing steps 1 & 2.

For an **Advanced-Level** balancing exercise, perform the beginner Kneeling Balance Board with your eyes closed.

AEROBIC & CARDIOVASCULAR EXERCISE

FEELING A BIT TIRED after your ride? Perhaps a little winded after climbing a flight of stairs? These are signs that you need to improve your endurance through aerobic exercise. Aerobic training affects your cardiorespiratory endurance by elevating your heart rate over an extended period of time. Here's how it works:

During sustained exercise your muscles depend upon oxygen to properly metabolize carbohydrates and fats into energy. Your heart pumps oxygenated blood to your muscles delivering the needed oxygen. When your heart is unable to keep up with your muscles' demand for oxygen you begin to experience fatigue. Consistent aerobic exercise turns your heart into a more efficient pumping mechanism by enabling it to pump more oxygenated blood with each stroke.

Consequently, aerobic training can combat fatigue and improve your energy level by increasing the rate at which your body can transport and utilize oxygen during exercise.

The key to aerobic exercise is to participate in a variety of activities. Varying your fitness routine will help you keep exercise fun and effective for the rest of your life. Choosing from aerobic activities such as walking, jogging, cycling, low-moderate impact aerobics classes, step bench, stair climbing, swimming, rowing, skating, and cross-country skiing can help keep you fit year-round in any climate. Another benefit from varying your exercises is that you receive a cross-training affect. This tunes your muscles to different movements and different intensities, resulting in less likelihood of injury, especially repetitive motion injuries, and in greater overall athleticism.

Here are some considerations concerning aerobic exercise:

■ To improve your cardiorespiratory endurance you should participate in an aerobic exercise at least 3 times a week and no more than 6 times a week. You can participate in aerobic activities on the same days you perform your strength-flexibility-balance workout or on alternate days.

■ Each aerobic workout should last between 30 to 45 minutes of continuous activity with your heart rate raised to your target level.

Monitoring Your Heart Rate

The intensity of your effort during exercise is a critical factor in improving your endurance and overall fitness. Your pace can be too fast or too slow. To receive the maximum aerobic benefit for your effort you should monitor your heartbeats-per-minute periodically during exercise and maintain your heart rate within 70%–85% of your maximum heart rate or lower (50%–60%) if you are interested in maximum "fat burning". This heart-rate zone is known as your exercise target zone. Consult the chart on the next page to determine your exercise target zone.

The most effective and reliable means of monitoring your exercise heart rate is with an electronic heart-rate monitor that attaches to your chest with an elastic belt. However, if you don't have access to a heart-rate monitor, you can manually count your heartbeats and

When you rest, your heart pumps an average of 5 liters of blood per minute. When you exercise, your muscles consume oxygen at a much faster rate, forcing your heart to pump faster and to pump more oxygenated blood per heartbeat ... up to an estimated 20 liters of blood per minute (or up to a whopping 30 liters per minute for an elite endurance athlete).

refer to the chart on the following page. Here are some key terms that will help you track your heart rate:

Aerobic target zone:

This is the heart rate zone that is most effective for receiving cardiorespiratory benefits.

Exercise heart rate:

Your "target" heart rate that is optimum for the benefits of aerobic exercise.

Fat-burning zone:

This is the heart rate zone that is most effective for "burning fat."

Maximum heart rate:

The maximum number of times your heart can contract in one minute.

Resting heart rate:

The number of heartbeats per minute when you are at complete rest.

Safety heart rate:

The heart rate suggested for beginner exercisers is 60% of their maximum heart rate. This is the minimum amount of stress you can place on your heart and still benefit from aerobic exercise.

Taking your heart rate:

As you exercise, periodically count your heartbeats for 15 seconds and multiply by 4. Refer to the chart to see if your heart rate is in your target zone. The trick to this is to not stop exercising while you monitor your heart rate. (If you stop, your heart rate immediately begins to fall and you will not get an accurate reading). If it falls below your target level, then you need to intensify your exercise effort. If it is above your target zone, then you are exercising too hard and you need to slow down.

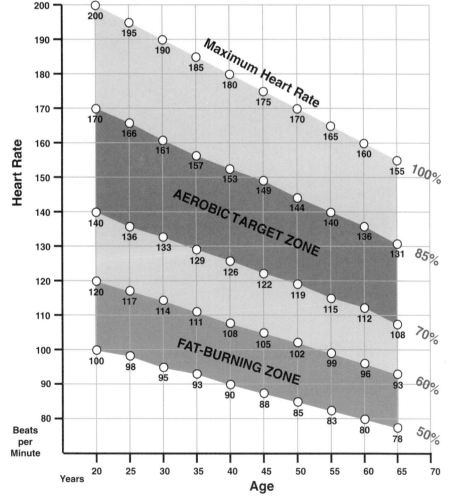

Your Exercise Target Heart Rate

Training Effect:
With consistent exercise your heart becomes a more efficient pump during periods of increased exertion. It pumps more blood with each stroke while your heart rate is reduced.

77

30-MINUTE WORKOUT

Adequate time is not always available. So, for those days when time is short, try this 30-minute workout. You will get a good basic workout on your most important muscles.

BEGINNER	INTERMEDIATE	ADVANCED
Warm-up	**Warm-up**	**Warm-up**
Crunches	Crunches	Crunches
Oblique Curl	Oblique Curl	5-Way Crunches
The Pointer	Prone Trunk Extension	The Advanced Pointer
Adductor Lift	Adductor-Quad Sets	Adductor-Quad Sets
The Squeeze	The Squeeze	The Squeeze
Theraband Fly	Theraband Fly	Prone Fly
Steeple	Steeple	Steeple
Angry Cat & Sway-back Horse	Angry Cat & Sway-back Horse	Angry Cat & Sway-back Horse
Runner's Stretch	Runner's Stretch	Runner's Stretch
Seated Ham Stretch	Seated Ham Stretch	Seated Ham Stretch
Sumo Stretch	Sumo Stretch	Sumo Stretch
Push-The-Wall-Down	Push-The-Wall-Down	Push-The-Wall-Down
Soleus Stretch	Soleus Stretch	Soleus Stretch

You can customize your workout by adding any exercises that address your personal needs and weaknesses.

45-MINUTE WORKOUT

When you have a little more time on your hands, try this 45-minute workout. You can customize your workout to fit your needs by including additional exercises that address your personal weaknesses.

BEGINNER	INTERMEDIATE	ADVANCED
Warm-up	**Warm-up**	**Warm-up**
Crunches	Crunches	Crunches
Oblique Curl	Oblique Curl	5-Way Crunches
The Pointer	Prone Trunk Extension	The Advanced Pointer
Adductor Lift	Adductor-Quad Sets	Adductor-Quad Sets
The Squeeze	The Squeeze	The Squeeze
Hamstring Curl	Hamstring Curl	Supine Leg Curl
Quad-Psoas Lift	Quad-Psoas Lift	Quad-Psoas Lift
Wall Pushes	Kneeling Push-Ups	Push-Ups
Theraband Fly	Theraband Fly	Prone Fly
Forward Arm Raise	Forward Arm Raise	Forward Arm Raise
Steeple	Steeple	Steeple
Dorsal Flex	Dorsal Flex	Dorsal Flex
Ventral Flex	Ventral Flex	Ventral Flex
Hip Stretch	Hip Stretch	Hip Stretch
Runner's Stretch	Runner's Stretch	Runner's Stretch
Seated Ham Stretch	Seated Ham Stretch	Seated Ham Stretch
Quad Stretch	Quad Stretch	Quad Stretch
Sumo Stretch	Sumo Stretch	Sumo Stretch
Push-The-Wall-Down	Push-The-Wall-Down	Push-The-Wall-Down
Soleus Stretch	Soleus Stretch	Soleus Stretch
Doorway Stretch	Doorway Stretch	Doorway Stretch
The Stork	The Stork	The Stork

60-MINUTE WORKOUT

The 60-minute workout is for those of you dedicated to reaching your full riding-fitness potential.

BEGINNER	INTERMEDIATE	ADVANCED
Warm-up	**Warm-up**	**Warm-up**
Crunches	Crunches	Crunches
Oblique Curl	Oblique Curl	5-Way Crunches
The Pointer	Prone Trunk Extension	The Advanced Pointer
Adductor Lift	Adductor Quad Sets	Adductor Quad Sets
The Squeeze	The Squeeze	The Squeeze
Hamstring Curl	Hamstring Curl	Supine Leg Curl
Quad-Psoas Lift	Quad-Psoas Lift	Quad-Psoas Lift
Heel Raise	Heel Raise	Heel Raise
Wall Pushes	Kneeling Push-Ups	Push-Ups
Theraband Fly	Theraband Fly	Prone Fly
Forward Arm Raise	Forward Arm Raise	Forward Arm Raise
Lateral Arm Raise	Lateral Arm Raise	Lateral Arm Raise
Kick-backs	Kick-backs	Overhead Extensions
Rotation Curl	Rotation Curl	Rotation Curl
Seat-specific Exercise	Seat-specific Exercise	Seat-specific Exercise
Orange Crush	Orange Crush	Orange Crush
Steeple	Steeple	Steeple
Dorsal Flex	Dorsal Flex	Dorsal Flex
Ventral Flex	Ventral Flex	Ventral Flex
Angry Cat & Sway-back Horse	Angry Cat & Sway-back Horse	Angry Cat & Sway-back Horse
Hip Stretch	Hip Stretch	Hip Stretch
Runner's Stretch	Runner's Stretch	Runner's Stretch
Seated Ham Stretch	Seated Ham Stretch	Seated Ham Stretch
Quad Stretch	Quad Stretch	Quad Stretch
Sumo Stretch	Sumo Stretch	Sumo Stretch
Push-The-Wall-Down	Push-The-Wall-Down	Push-The-Wall-Down
Soleus Stretch	Soleus Stretch	Soleus Stretch
Doorway Stretch	Doorway Stretch	Doorway Stretch
Reach-For-The-Sky	Reach-For-The-Sky	Reach-For-The-Sky
The Stork	The Stork	The Stork
Kneeling Balance Board	Kneeling Balance Board	Kneeling Balance Board

THE *NEW* TOTAL RIDER

2

The Nutrition Advantage

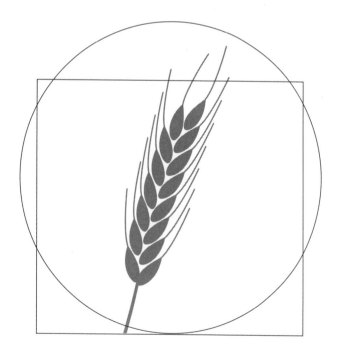

THE NUTRITION ADVANTAGE

Creating Energetic Balance with Food: An Ayurvedic Perspective with Pilar Martin

OBVIOUSLY THERE ARE DIETS out there that are healthy and beneficial. However, the questions on most of our minds seem to be these : Is there an easy way of being healthy? Is there a healthy lifestyle that I can actually pursue comfortably and confidently? And, since I'm an active equestrian, can this nutritional lifestyle improve my performance in riding and exercise?

The answer to these questions is a resounding yes! There is a healthy nutritional lifestyle called Ayurveda that feels natural and instinctive, delivers remarkable results and will benefit your overall well-being and your athletic-equestrian endeavors. To further explain, **The New Total Rider** turned to Pilar Martin, Ayurvedic and nutritional expert.

CREATE A HEALTHY LIFESTYLE

A healthy diet will supply you with fuel for energy, regulators for life-processes, and building materials for growth, maintenance and repair. These life-long nutritional needs are fulfilled with vital nutrients such as water, carbohydrates (including fiber), fats, proteins, vitamins and minerals. Ideally your eating lifestyle will provide balanced and sufficient amounts of these nutrients, generate only the amount of energy you require to maintain your appropriate weight and body composition, offer a variety of foods that fit your tastes, family and cultural traditions, and budget.

The typical American diet, for example, falls far short of these goals, Americans as a group still eat too much protein, fat, salt and sugar, and not enough carbohydrates, fiber and water found in fresh, vital foods. As a result, we are a culture that puts up with less than optimal health and relies heavily on pharmaceuticals to resolve health issues.

It is now known that our genes dictate up to one-third of the diseases we get due to aging, while the way we live is responsible for the other two-thirds. This means that creating vibrant health and maximum performance can largely, and for a limited time, be a matter of choice. You can dramatically affect your health, energy and athletic performance through the lifestyle choices you make every day.

Here are 4 powerful steps to creating a healthy lifestyle and building the foundation for optimal performance:

1. Eat fresh foods.

Fresh food goes beyond being merely ripe. When you eat a tomato recently picked from your garden, notice the difference from the tomatoes you buy at the supermarket. That difference can be described in terms of taste, smell, feel and appearance, but there is something extra. That tomato from your garden is still full of vitality. It is full of life. When you slice it and eat it, you can taste and feel its life energy. That epitomizes the definition of fresh. Fresh food is food that imparts abundant nutrients, vital energy and life to you. You receive the vitality of the food as a living organism when you eat it. It is this vitality that fully supports your well-being. Therefore, choosing fresh food involves considering its vital energy as well as its ripeness. Look for food that is rich in both nutrients and vital life energy.

If you don't have a garden, then how do you find the freshest food? You can shop at your local farmer's markets during growing seasons, or at local health food stores. You can even find truly fresh food at the supermarkets if you are willing to ask a few questions to determine the quality of the food you're buying. These 3 questions can help you find the freshest food available:

▮ Was it grown locally or regionally?

83

■ Is this its natural season?

■ How long has it been since it was harvested?

As a rule, the fresher a food is, the less processed it is, and the less processed a food is, the healthier it is for you. Wherever possible, cook with and eat fresh, unprocessed foods instead of their more refined or processed counterparts. Eat apples instead of drinking apple juice, or use fresh tomatoes in your marinara, instead of canned tomato paste. Eat breads and pastas that use whole grains in their ingredients instead of highly processed white flour.

2. Eat organic foods.

Organic foods are grown with techniques that utilize healthy soil, air and water. Organically grown plants do not require applications of herbicides, pesticides, fungicides and synthetic fertilizers or other artificial support in order to thrive. The basic principle is the healthier the soil is, the more nutrients and energy it provides to the plants growing in it. As a result of these superior growing techniques, organically grown foods are stronger and provide consumers with greater quantity of quality nutrients and vital life energy.

Commercially grown food, on the other hand, is grown with the aid of synthetic chemicals and places significantly less measurable nutrients and energy on your dinner plate. However, you do ingest dramatically higher levels of toxins.

The argument for eating organic foods is straightforward and simple. Don't put ineffective, toxic fuel into your bodies. If you want to feel and perform like a racecar, then treat yourself like a Ferrari, not a junker. Use only the best fuel you can find. When you build your eating lifestyle around fresh, whole, organic food, you will minimize the amount of toxins, and maximize the amount and quality of nutrients and energy ingested into your body. Eating toxin-free, nutrient-rich, energy-rich food is a simple and sensible method to place you squarely on the path to vibrant health.

3. Eat more high quality carbohydrates and less protein.

Diets that are rich in high quality, natural carbohydrates and low in protein have formed the nutritional foundation for all recorded healthy, long-lived cultures. In his book, **Conscious Eating**, Gabriel Cousens, M.D. states, "It is a well established fact that the longest-lived people throughout the world, such as the Hunzkuts, Bulgarians, East Indian Todas, Russian Caucasians and Yucatan Indians, are either complete vegetarians or eat meat infrequently. They eat between one third to one half the protein that we eat in the U.S."

Protein is necessary for the proper functioning of our bodies; however, moderating the protein in your diet by eating less meat, poultry, seafood and fewer dairy products, can provide numerous benefits to your overall health and well being, as well as your athletic performance, such as:

Reducing the risk of common nutritionally-related diseases such as hypertension, heart disease, atherosclerosis, kidney damage, arthritis, and various forms of cancer, etc.

Reducing the risk of osteoporosis. According to overwhelming evidence, the most important step you can take to prevent osteoporosis is to lower the amount of protein in your diet. One of the consequences of high protein diets is calcium loss from your bones, which produces a loss in bone density. Numerous research studies on the relationship of vegetarianism and osteoporosis have shown that vegetarian women can have significantly less bone loss (up to 5 times less) than non-vegetarian women by the age of 65. It is common knowledge that when body builders begin their extreme high protein diets to prepare for competition, they supplement massive amounts of minerals in an attempt to offset the dramatic loss of calcium and other minerals. However, high calcium supplementation does not seem to make a significant difference in the prevention or treatment of osteoporosis. Dr. Cousens also relates this observation: "The Bantus, an African tribe, get about 350 mg of calcium per day, almost one fourth of the National Dairy Council recommendation. The Bantu women, however, do not suffer from osteoporosis and rarely suffer from bone fractures. Although there may be some genetic component helping the Bantus, it is significant that the genetic relatives of the Bantus in the U.S., who are eating the standard American diet, have bone loss percentages that are about the same as the U.S. Caucasian population."

Moderating the protein in your diet will increase your endurance and recovery time after exercise. A vegetarian diet typically doubles a person's endurance level. Numerous world-class and Olympic athletes have chosen low meat or vegetarian diets for the proven endurance and recovery benefits.

Switching from a diet of refined, high protein foods to a healthier diet with quality nutrients and moderate protein has also been shown to elevate feelings of calm and patience, and decrease feelings of anxiety, stress and aggression. Consider what this could mean for your own sense of well-being, your relationships with other people, and your interactions with your horse. The implications of increased patience and calm for your training, competitive performance and enjoyment of the sport could be astounding.

4. Create nutritional and energetic balance.

A system that is proven to create balance in an easy and natural way is the science of Ayurveda. Think of it as an owner's manual to your body that guides you in staying healthy and enjoying life to its full potential. Once implemented into your lifestyle, the principles of Ayurveda will powerfully affect your health, your relationships and your entire environment.

Ayurveda is based on the premise that the body, mind and spirit are aspects of a whole being ... you, and therefore cannot be divided when you address your health. When all three aspects are in balance and function at their optimum potential, you experience vibrant health, happiness and your true nature. If one or more of the three aspects of body, mind and spirit becomes out of balance with the others, then your whole being suffers and becomes vulnerable to disease and illness. The guiding premise of Ayurveda is simple: Have your whole being operate optimally by keeping the elements of your being in balance.

Consider that you are born with a particular combination of five elements: Ether (Space), Air, Fire, Water and Earth. In fact, everything in nature is comprised of all 5 of these essential elements. There are a number of different combinations and each one produces specific characteristics. Your combination of elements determines what you are and the way you are. Each element has certain qualities that will either aggravate or reduce a certain condition. Air, for instance, is drying and has a drying effect. Water has a moistening effect, Fire has a heating effect, and Earth has a structuring effect. When you add an element and its corresponding effect, then its opposite will diminish, so you add the element that is opposite to the aggravated condition in order to balance it. It is precisely these five elements that you are striving to keep in balance in order to maintain an optimal state of health and well being.

However, the changes that occur in life, whether through nature, by accident, or self-induced, can throw off this unique balance. So, in the face of life's circumstances, how do you keep yourself in balance? And how can you simplify this approach to make it easily manageable?

The first step is to identify your own particular physical and mental combinations of elements by identifying your type or "dosha." You can identify your primary dosha(s) in this book by completing the questionnaire that begins on the following page. All of the elements and their possible combinations have been condensed into three types or "doshas" known as Vata, Pitta and Kapha:

Vata = ether and air
Pitta = water and fire
Kapha = water and earth

You may exhibit one dosha stronger than the other two:

V3	P1	K1
V1	P3	K1
V1	P1	K3

For example, if you exhibit the Pitta dosha stronger than the other two, then you are "Pitta." If you exhibit Kapha stronger than Vata or Pitta, than you are "Kapha."

Or, you may exhibit two doshas stronger than the third:

V3	P3	K1
V1	P3	K3
V3	P1	K3

If you exhibit Vata and Pitta much stronger than Kapha, then you are "Vata-Pitta." Or, you may exhibit all three doshas in equal amounts:

| V3 | P3 | K3 |

In this case, you are "Tri-doshic."

The combination of elements you are born with is perfect for you, so you don't need to wonder which dosha is better. You only need to know which of your doshas is out of balance and how can you bring it back into balance.

QUESTIONNAIRE

SECTION 1

Check the 1 or 2 statements in each category that best describe your physical characteristics.

PHYSICAL TRAITS	VATA CONSTITUTION	PITTA CONSTITUTION	KAPHA CONSTITUTION
FRAME	I am thin, lanky and slender with prominent joints and thin muscles. ❑	I have a medium symmetrical build with good muscle development ❑	I have a large, round or stocky build. My frame is broad, stout or thick. ❑
WEIGHT	Low; I may forget to eat or have a tendency to lose weight. ❑	Moderate; it is easy for me to gain or lose weight if I put my mind to it. ❑	Heavy; I gain weight easily and have difficulty losing it. ❑
EYES	My eyes are small and active. ❑	I have a penetrating gaze. ❑	I have large pleasant eyes. ❑
COMPLEXION	My skin is dry, rough or thin. ❑	My skin is warm, reddish in color and prone to irritation. ❑	My skin is thick, moist and smooth. ❑
HAIR	My hair is dry, brittle or frizzy. ❑	My hair is fine with a tendency towards early thinning or graying. ❑	I have abundant, thick and oily hair. ❑
JOINTS	My joints are thin and prominent and have a tendency to crack. ❑	My joints are loose and flexible. ❑	My joints are large, well knit and padded. ❑
SLEEP PATTERN	I am a light sleeper with a tendency to awaken easily. ❑	I am a moderately sound sleeper; I usually need less than 8 hours to feel rested. ❑	My sleep is deep and long. I tend to awaken slowly in the morning. ❑
BODY TEMPERATURE	My hands and feet are usually cold and I prefer warm environments. ❑	I am usually warm, regardless of the season, and prefer cooler environments. ❑	I am adaptable to most temperatures but do not like cold, wet days. ❑
TEMPERAMENT	I am lively and enthusiastic by nature. ❑	I am purposeful and intense. I like to convince. ❑	I am easy-going and accepting. I like to support. ❑
UNDER STRESS	I become anxious and/or worried. ❑	I become irritable and/or aggressive. ❑	I become withdrawn and/or reclusive. ❑
SECTION 1 TOTAL:	VATA =	PITTA =	KAPHA =

87

SECTION 2

Using the following scale, indicate how each statement applies to your life experiences over the past 30 to 60 days:

		Not at all	Slightly	Somewhat	Moderately	Very
1.	I have been feeling worried or anxious.	1	2	3	4	5
2.	I've been having difficulty falling asleep or have been awakening easily.	1	2	3	4	5
3.	I feel restless if I'm not constantly on the move.	1	2	3	4	5
4.	My digestion is irregular with frequent gas or bloating.	1	2	3	4	5
5.	My bowel movements are hard, dry or occur less than once per day.	1	2	3	4	5
6.	My daily schedule of eating meals, going to sleep or awakening often varies from day to day.	1	2	3	4	5
7.	I tend to be impulsive.	1	2	3	4	5
8.	I often forget things after a short period of time.	1	2	3	4	5
9.	I have a lot of initiative, but have trouble following through.	1	2	3	4	5
10.	I generally have a number of physical concerns.	1	2	3	4	5

Vata Score = _____

		Not at all	Slightly	Somewhat	Moderately	Very
1.	I have been feeling irritable or impatient.	1	2	3	4	5
2.	I tend to be critical and am intolerant of errors.	1	2	3	4	5
3.	My skin feels hot and irritated, or breaks out easily.	1	2	3	4	5
4.	I have been having acid indigestion or heartburn.	1	2	3	4	5
5.	I tend to be compulsive and have difficulty stopping once I've started a project.	1	2	3	4	5
6.	I am easily frustrated by other people's incompetence.	1	2	3	4	5

	Not at all	Slightly	Somewhat	Moderately	Very
7. Spicy foods, while I might enjoy them, usually do not agree with me.	1	2	3	4	5
8. I am strongly opinionated and tend to share my point of view without being asked.	1	2	3	4	5
9. I often feel as if I am overheated or have a low-grade fever.	1	2	3	4	5
10. When provoked, I can be sarcastic or biting.	1	2	3	4	5

Pitta Score = _____

	Not at all	Slightly	Somewhat	Moderately	Very
1. I am currently overweight and have difficulty losing extra pounds.	1	2	3	4	5
2. I have a slow digestion and feel heavy after eating.	1	2	3	4	5
3. I commonly experience sinus congestion or excessive phlegm in my respiratory tract.	1	2	3	4	5
4. I continue to remain in a relationship, even though it is no longer nourishing.	1	2	3	4	5
5. I often deal with conflict by withdrawing.	1	2	3	4	5
6. I easily accumulate clutter in my life.	1	2	3	4	5
7. I have difficulty getting going in the morning.	1	2	3	4	5
8. I like to maintain a routine and resist changing my pace.	1	2	3	4	5
9. Given a choice, I prefer to watch rather than participate in an athletic activity.	1	2	3	4	5
10. I regularly feel drowsy or sluggish after a meal.	1	2	3	4	5

Kapha Score = _____

Totals for Section 1:	Vata =	Pitta =	Kapha =
Totals for Section 2:	Vata =	Pitta =	Kapha =

Interpreting Your Results

Section 1 is an inquiry into the proportion of each of the 3 principle doshas within your unique mind-body constitution. Your score in this section reflects your basic nature. These characteristics tend to change very slowly over your lifetime.

The principle that received the highest number of checks is the most predominant force in your overall mind-body make-up. The principle that received the next highest number of checks is the secondary force in your constitution. The lowest scoring principle, while still an active force in your mind-body physiology, is the least dominant in your particular constitution.

Section 2 provides a snapshot of your current mind-body state. The mind-body dosha that scores the highest number of points is the one requiring the most attention at this time. A score of 30 points or higher in any section also indicates the potential need for balancing.

Now, let's see what the Vata, Pitta and Kapha doshas are all about.

Vata is responsible for any and all movement in your body and mind, and any space in your body. Examples include perspiration, circulation and excretion. Vata is very closely associated with sound, since sound travels in air.

Pitta is responsible for all transformation that takes place in your body and mind, especially the conversion of food into nutrients, the intake of energy through your eyes and the interpretations your mind gives to both. It also governs your digestive enzymes and the continuous transformation of light into energy. Sight is closely associated with Pitta, since fire gives light.

Kapha is responsible for all lubrication, cohesiveness and stability in your body and mind. This includes your fluids, muscles, bones, endurance and stability of mind. Taste is closely associated with Kapha.

The key to keeping yourself in a healthy balance is to live a lifestyle that naturally balances your doshas, and when you are out of balance, eat foods and make other adjustments that supply you with the elements you need to regain balance. This process is relatively easy and it integrates simply and naturally into your lifestyle once you understand the principle of maintaining balance. You can determine what is needed in any moment by noticing your physical, mental and emotional states, and by being aware of your natural rhythms and the effects foods have on you.

Follow Your Natural Rhythms

Think of your environment as your extended body. You are always interacting with your environment, and it with you; in fact, there is not a single moment when you don't exchange something with it. You breathe your environment in and breathe yourself out in a constant melding of both. This intimate relationship with your environment is crucial to your well-being, and it demands awareness and maintenance of the inherent natural balance.

The first step in maintaining your natural balance is to become aware of the rhythms of nature that support you in experiencing vibrant natural health. You are a part of nature to the degree that the rhythms of nature are your own intrinsic rhythms. These larger cycles do not occur separate from you. They are your own internal rhythms that influence your mental, emotional and physical well being in identifiable ways; for example, when you lose touch with your body's rhythms, you experience discomfort or fatigue. Some of the known rhythms of nature include:

- **Circadian rhythms**: 24-hour cycle of night and day

- **Seasonal rhythms:** 12-month cycle of Spring, Summer, Autumn, Winter

90

■ **Lunar rhythms**: Monthly cycle of moon revolving around earth.

■ **Tidal rhythms**: Gravitational influence of the moon on the waters of the earth.

Since the rhythms of nature are also your own internal rhythms, following these larger cycles simply means taking the time to listen to your body and to incorporate some basic steps in your daily routine that will help you care for yourself. You don't have to memorize tidal charts from around the globe. When you are aware of your own natural rhythms, you can choose to adjust your lifestyle so that it fully supports your well-being and happiness. Here are several adaptations that help you maintain your natural balance by being in harmony with the changing seasons. Like most of the recommendations in Ayurveda, they are common-sense suggestions and simple to implement:

Spring = Wet, cold months
Favor lighter, warmer foods and spices. Stay warm and dry.

Summer = Warm months
Choose activities, foods and clothing that will keep you cool.

Autumn & Winter: = Dry, cold months
Keep your skin lubricated, choose warmer and heavier foods such as hearty soups, stews and casseroles.

Examine your daily routine and how your energy and feelings shift throughout the day. How you feel physically, emotionally, etc. is influenced by your daily circadian rhythms. There are certain times of each day when you naturally have more energy, just as there are specific times when your digestion is naturally stronger. Notice how you experience fluctuations during the course of a day. Look for opportunities to make simple adjustments to provide balance and positively influence your well-being.

Experiment with the following suggestions for adapting your daily routine to be in sync with your circadian rhythms and see how they influence the quality of your life:

Morning: 6:00 a.m.–10:00 a.m.

■ Wake up and drink a warm glass of water. This signals your digestive system to eliminate toxins.

■ Empty your bowels and bladder.

■ Clean your teeth, tongue, and gums.

■ Massage your body with natural, unprocessed oil. This nourishes your tissues, stimulates your skin to release health-promoting chemicals, improves your circulation, increases alertness, facilitates detoxification and strengthens your immune system. Use sesame oil for vata constitutions, coconut or sunflower for pitta, and a small amount of safflower, mustard, or almond oil for a stimulating massage for kapha.

■ Bathe.

■ Do flexibility exercises such as yoga postures or stretching.

■ Meditate or simply sit quietly and watch your thoughts without getting into them.

■ Eat a very light breakfast (if you're hungry). Be aware of what you're eating, how you're eating and how your food choice will affect you.

■ Morning work and activity.

Midday: Noon–1:00 p.m.

■ Eat lunch. Make it the largest meal of the day.

■ Sit quietly for a few minutes after eating.

■ Walk 5–15 minutes to aid your digestion.

91

Evening: 6:00–7:00 p.m.

- Sit quietly or meditate for at least 20 minutes after your afternoon work and activity.

- Eat a light dinner.

- Sit quietly a few minutes afterwards.

- Walk 5–15 minutes.

Ideal sleeping time: 10:00 p.m.–6:00 a.m.

- This is a time for light activity. Minimize reading, eating or watching T.V. Your body rejuvenates at this time by digesting left-over toxins.

- Try to be in bed with lights out by 10:30.

10:00 p.m.–2:00 a.m.
Your physical body rejuvenates.

2:00 a.m.–6:00 am.
Dream. Your emotional body rejuvenates.

You also want to pay particular attention to times of change in your life, because major changes can be stressful and may provoke imbalances. During these times you want to maintain your habits of good health, including meditation, regular exercise, sensory nourishment, and emotional healing. When you are feeling stressed, simplify your diet and favor the following foods to help restore balance to your physiology:

- Locally-grown fruits and vegetables

- Homemade soups, broths, stews

- Fresh juices

- Easily-digested foods, e.g. steamed rice and vegetables

And avoid these foods:

- Frozen, canned and pre-packaged foods

- Fermented foods and drinks

- Aged cheeses

- Leftovers

- Highly refined foods

The Effects of Foods

You can use foods to help maintain your natural balance. When you are out of balance certain foods can help you to restore balance, while other foods will further aggravate your imbalance.

All foods have specific qualities that cause you to exhibit certain physical and emotional effects. For example, a sweet food will increase Kapha and decrease Pitta and Vata. To help you understand how what you eat affects your well-being, Ayurveda identifies six tastes inherent in foods and their effects in your system:

Sweet:	↓V	↓P	↑K
Sour:	↓V	↑P	↓K
Salty:	↓V	↑P	↑K
Bitter:	↑V	↓P	↓K
Pungent:	↑V	↑P	↓K
Astringent:	↑V	↓P	↓K

(↑ = increases, ↓ = decreases)

Each taste has identifiable physical effects:

TASTE	PHYSICAL EFFECTS	COMMON SOURCES
Sweet	Most nutritive; builds body tissue	Sugar, honey, milk, butter, rice, breads, pastas, meats (carbohydrates, fats, proteins)
Sour	Improves appetite and digestion; promotes digestion	Citrus fruits, yogurt, cheese, tomatoes, salad dressings, pickles, vinegar (organic acids)
Salty	Mildly laxative/sedative; promotes digestion	Salt, sauces, salted meats, fish (mineral salt)
Pungent	Stimulates digestion Clears congestion	Hot peppers, salsa, ginger, radishes, Mustard greens, cloves, horseradish (essential oils)
Bitter	Anti-inflammatory Detoxifying	Green leafy vegetables, eggplant, radishes, celery, sprouts, beets, (alkaloids, glycosides)
Astringent	Drying; compacts system	Beans, tea, apples, pomegranates, Cauliflower, dark leafy greens (tannins)

The six tastes also directly affect enzyme production in your digestive system. Even the emotional effects of the six tastes are identified:

TASTE	BALANCED	OUT OF BALANCE
Sweet	nurturing	cloying
Sour	stimulating	caustic
Salty	earthy	hedonistic
Pungent	passionate	hostile
Bitter	disciplined	resentful
Astringent	witty	cynical

If your diet includes all six tastes on a regular basis, with preference given to those tastes that benefit your constitution, then your body will be able to digest everything you eat and stay in balance. You do not need to count calories, serving quantities or keep track of lists.

Balancing Foods For Each Dosha

The following Dosha Food Charts were developed according to guidelines given by Ayurvedic physician Dr. Robert Svoboda. The charts list the foods that are generally balancing and unbalancing for each dosha. Use these charts as general guidelines, not as rigid rules. Discover for yourself which guidelines are important to follow and which can be safely ignored on occasion. Allow yourself time to become comfortable with your individual guidelines, and in the process, learn to listen attentively to your body and mind. Pay close attention to what you eat and how you feel after your meal. Experiment with individual food choices; for example, observe how bananas affect you over the course of a day or a week. Learn the basic principles and guidelines and then play and enjoy fine tuning your lifestyle. You will eventually become very astute about how your food choices and your environment affect how you feel, and you will become the best barometer of how balanced or unbalanced you are in a given moment.

FOODS FOR VATA

Sweet, sour and **salty** foods are generally **balancing** for Vata. They are satisfying and minimize insecurity about being well fed.

Bitter, pungent and **astringent** foods are **unbalancing** for Vata, since they are drying and intensify emotional instability, especially insecurity. Vata is also aggravated by excess of any particular food or taste, so avoid large amounts.

Grains	**Oats, Rice** and **Wheat** are balancing for Vata when well-cooked. **Unyeasted Bread** is more balancing than yeasted bread.
	Buckwheat, Corn, Millet and **Rye** can be drying, so only eat occasionally for variety, and add butter, ghee or oil to reduce dryness. **Yeasted Bread** is unbalancing for Vata, since it is filled with gas after fermentation.
Vegetables	**Asparagus, Beets, Carrots, Celery, Garlic, Green Beans, Okra, Onion, Parsnips, Radishes, Rutabagas, Turnips, Sweet Potatoes** and **Water Chestnuts** are balancing when well-cooked. In general, **cooked vegetables** are more balancing to Vata than raw vegetables. Rough, hard vegetables such as celery are better ingested as a juice.
	Cucumbers, Eggplant, Mushrooms, Peas, Spinach, Squashes and **Zucchini** can be eaten occasionally for variety if well-cooked in oil. **Tomatoes** are suitable on occasion when cooked, and the skin and seeds are removed. **Cilantro, Parsley, Lettuce, Spinach** and **Sprouts** are suitable on occasion if eaten with a good oily or creamy dressing.
	In general, **raw vegetables** are unbalancing for Vata. Vatas whose joints ache and feel stiff should avoid **Spinach, Potatoes, Tomatoes, Eggplant** and **Peppers**.
Fruits	**Apricots** and **Mangoes** are especially good for Vata. **Avocados, Berries, Cherries, Coconut, Dates, Figs, Grapefruit, Grapes, Lemons, Nectarines, Oranges, Papaya, Peaches, Pears, Persimmons, Pineapples** and **Plums** are all balancing for Vata when ripe.
	Bananas and **Melons** should be eaten in moderation.
	Astringent fruits like **Cranberries** and **Pomegranates**, and drying fruits like **Apples** are unbalancing for Vata. **Unripe fruits** and **dried fruits** are also unbalancing.
Flesh Foods	Vatas are the only people who need animal foods (for the complete proteins) in their diets; however, moderation is still the rule, since overindulgence quickly weakens Vata digestion.

95

Chicken, Turkey, Fresh Fish, Goat and **Venison** are generally good when eaten in moderation.
Lamb and **Beef** can be eaten on rare occasion.
Eggs are balancing if scrambled or poached.

Lamb and **Beef** should not be eaten regularly.
Shellfish should be avoided because of its potential to cause allergies.
Fried Eggs are unbalancing and should be avoided.

Legumes	Vatas should ingest only small amounts of legumes at any one meal. **Legumes**, like meat, are high in hard-to-digest proteins and produce nitrogenous waste by-products, which unbalance Vata. Increased Vata due to beans and peas usually occurs as intestinal gas. Reduce the gas-producing qualities by soaking the legumes in water for at least an hour, and then change the water. To further reduce the possibility of gas, you can boil them in the fresh water for 5-10 minutes and then throw out that water before completing cooking.
	Black Lentils, Red Lentils, Chickpeas, Mung Beans and **Tofu** are good when eaten in moderation. **Mung Beans** are the best because they are the easiest to digest. Split peas and split lentils are also easier to digest.
	Try cooking beans and peas with turmeric, cumin, coriander, ginger or garlic to help prevent your Vata from being aggravated.
	Peanuts can contribute to blood clotting and should be avoided by anyone who has impaired circulation.
Nuts and Seeds	**All Nuts** and **Seeds** are balancing for Vata when eaten occasionally in moderation. Regular consumption can cause indigestion. However, **Nut Butters** and **Seed Butters** can be eaten regularly.
	Almonds are considered to be the best of the nuts. Always soak them overnight, and then peel them before eating. The skins can be irritating so never eat them with their skins on.
Oils	**All oils** are good for Vata. **Sesame Oil** is the best for Vata and **Safflower Oil** is the least beneficial. Try **Coconut** and **Sesame Oils** for your hair, and **Mustard Oil** for your skin.
Dairy	**All dairy products** are considered to be good for those Vatas who are not allergic to them. However, **hard cheeses** are very concentrated and should be eaten sparingly.
Sweeteners	Vatas can use any **sweetener** in moderation except white sugar, which is poisonous for them. **Honey** should never be cooked.
Spices	**All spices**, especially **Garlic** and **Ginger** are good for Vatas in small quantities. Vatas are often tempted to overuse spices, but too much of any spice can become aggravating, so keep your seasonings in moderation.

FOODS FOR PITTA

Sweet, bitter and **astringent** foods are cooling and balancing for the naturally "hot" Pitta, while **sour, salty** and **pungent** foods are heating and unbalancing. **Grains, fruits** and **vegetables** should form the bulk of the Pitta diet. **Meat, eggs, alcohol** and **salt** should be avoided or minimized, as these foods augment Pitta's natural compulsive tendencies and aggressiveness. Pitta people benefit the most from a **vegetarian** lifestyle.

Grains	**Barley** is the best for Pittas, as it cools, dries and helps to reduce excess stomach acid. **Rice, Oats** and **Wheat** are also balancing. **Unyeasted Breads** are balancing for Pitta.
	Buckwheat, Corn, Millet and **Rye** are heating and should not be eaten regularly. **Yeasted Bread** is unbalancing for Pitta due to its sourness, produced during fermentation.
Vegetables	**Asparagus, Broccoli, Brussels Sprouts, Cabbage, Cilantro, Cucumber, Cauliflower, Celery, Cress, Green Beans, Leafy Greens, Lettuce, Mushrooms, Okra, Peas, Parsley, Potatoes, Sprouts, Squashes, Water Chestnuts** and **Zucchini** are all especially balancing for Pitta.
	Beets, Carrots and **Daikon Radishes** can be beneficial and eaten occasionally as long as your Pitta is not already aggravated. **Steamed White** or **Yellow Onions** can be good on occasion because they become sweet and lose their pungency when cooked. **Vegetables not on the list** can be good when they are unusually sweet.
	Pittas can eat a wide variety of vegetables and should be primarily concerned with avoiding **Sour** and **Pungent** vegetables. Avoid **Tomatoes** in all forms. Pungent vegetables like **Garlic, Red** and **Purple Onions, Peppers** and **Radishes** should also be avoided.
Fruits	**Apples, Apricots, Avocados, Cherries, Coconut, Dried Fruits, Figs, Grapes, Lemons, Mangoes, Melons, Nectarines, Oranges, Peaches, Pears, Persimmons, Pineapples, Plums** and **Pomegranates** are all balancing for Pittas when they are sweet. **Mangoes, Figs** and **Grapes** are especially good for Pittas.
	Any fruit, including those on the balancing list, should not be eaten by Pittas if it is sour. Likewise, **fruit not on this list** can be eaten if it is exceptionally sweet. **Lemons** and **Limes** are normally sour, however, they can be balancing for Pittas if used sparingly and overuse is avoided.

97

Bananas are sweet, however, they have a sour post-digestive effect and should not be eaten regularly by Pittas.
Papaya is also sweet, but is too "hot" for Pittas' already blazing constitution and should be avoided.

Flesh Foods	**Chicken, Turkey, Rabbit** and **Venison** are permissible for Pittas. **Egg whites** are cooling if eaten in moderation.
	Even though Pittas can digest flesh foods, they should generally avoid them since they pollute Pittas' blood and promote aggression and irritability. Avoid all **Seafood**, which is too "hot" and can cause allergies in Pittas. Also avoid **Egg Yolks**, which are heating.
Legumes	**Black Lentils, Chickpeas, Mung Beans, Tofu** and most other legumes are good for Pittas if eaten in small quantities.
	Red and **Yellow Lentils** are unbalancing and should be avoided.
Nuts and Seeds	**Coconut, Sunflower Seeds**, and **Pumpkinseeds** are balancing. **Fresh Coconut Milk** is especially good for Pittas.
	Avoid most **other nuts and seeds**, as they are too hot and oily for Pittas.
Oils	Pittas can use **Coconut, Olive** and **Sunflower Oils**, and smaller amounts of **Almond** and **Flax Oils**; however, excessive consumption of oils of any kind should be avoided.
Dairy	**Milk, Unsalted Butter, Ghee** and other sweet dairy products are good in moderation. Pittas should stick with **Soft, Unsalted Cheeses**.
	Sour dairy products such as **Yogurt** and **Hard Cheeses** should be avoided. **Yogurt** can be eaten in small amounts if it is sweetened, spiced with cinnamon or coriander and a few drops of lemon, then blended with an equal part water.
Sweeteners	**Sweets** reduce heat and can relieve aggravated Pitta. Out of all the doshas, Pittas can best handle sweets, including **Sugar**. **Honey** is good in small-to-moderate quantities. In fact, Pittas do well with almost all **Sweeteners** in moderation.
	Here's the exception: **Molasses** is too hot for Pittas and should be avoided.
Spices	**Cooling spices** such as **Cardamom, Cinnamon, Coriander, Fennel,** and **Turmeric** are best for Pittas. Small amounts of **Black Pepper** are good. A small amount of **Cumin** is okay if mixed with **Coriander**.
	Most spices are heating and increase Pitta aggressiveness. **Mustard** and **Salt** in particular should be eliminated from the Pitta diet. Avoid other hot spices.

FOODS FOR KAPHA

Bitter, Pungent and **Astringent** foods are balancing for Kaphas, and invigorate their bodies and minds. Kaphas benefit from eating plenty of **vegetables** and limiting the total amount of food they consume. Kaphas should avoid **Sweet, Sour** and **Salty** foods. Also avoid **fried**, or otherwise **greasy foods, dairy products** and **fat in general**.

Grains	Kaphas need less grain than Vatas and Pittas. Hot, drying grains such as **Buckwheat** and **Millet** are best, followed by **Barley, Rice** and **Corn**. Grains should be eaten roasted or dry-cooked.
	Breads should be toasted and eaten sparingly. Better yet, avoid Breads altogether.
	Wheat should be avoided, as it is too heavy, cold and oily for Kaphas.
Vegetables	**Most vegetables** are good for Kaphas; in fact, eat as many vegetables as you like as often as you like. **Leafy Greens** and **Vegetables with seeds**, like **Squashes** and **Peppers**, are preferable over **Root Vegetables**. **Raw vegetables** are good; however, **steamed vegetables** are easier to digest.
	Potatoes, Tomatoes and **Water Chestnuts** are unbalancing for Kaphas and should be avoided.
Fruits	**Apples, Apricots, Cranberries, Mangoes, Peaches, Pears** and **Pomegranates** are best. **Dried fruits**, such as **Prunes**, are good for Kaphas.
	Avoid very sweet, very sour and very juicy fruits.
Flesh Foods	Kaphas rarely need flesh foods because they are adequately nourished by other foods; however, they can eat **Chicken, Eggs, Rabbit, Seafood** and **Venison** in moderation. Flesh foods should be roasted, broiled, baked or grilled.
Legumes	Legumes are better than meat for Kaphas, due to the lack of animal fat. The best legumes are **Black Beans, Mung Beans, Pinto Beans** and **Red Lentils**. Well-cooked **Tofu** is okay in small quantities.
	Avoid heavy legumes such as **Black Lentils, Kidney Beans** and **Soybeans**.
Nuts and Seeds	**Nuts** and **Seeds** are heavy and oily and should be avoided. **Sunflower Seeds** and **Pumpkin Seeds** can be eaten on occasion.
Oils	In general, avoid using oils; however, Kaphas may use **Almond, Corn, Safflower** or **Sunflower Oils** when necessary.
Dairy	**Goat's Milk** is better for Kaphas since it is "hotter" and lighter for digestion than cow's milk, and does not promote respiratory diseases. **Ghee** is good in small amounts.

Dairy products have heavy, oily, sticky and cooling qualities and should be avoided.

Sweeteners	Avoid **Sweets**, except for **Raw Honey**, which helps reduce Kapha imbalance.
Spices	Kaphas can use almost all Spices. **Ginger** and **Garlic** are best.
	Avoid **Salt**. It increases Kapha imbalance.

CREATING BALANCE WITH FOOD: A QUICK REFERENCE

	To Reduce Vata Air Element Choose **warm**, **oily**, **heavy** foods, and **sweet**, **sour**, **salty** tastes.	To Reduce Pitta Fire Element Choose **cool** foods and liquids, and **sweet**, **bitter**, **astringent** tastes.	To Reduce Kapha Earth Element Choose **light**, **dry**, warm foods, & **pungent**, **bitter**, **astringent** tastes.
Dairy	**Favor** all dairy. Eat hard cheeses sparingly.	**Favor** milk, butter, and ghee. **Reduce** yogurt, cheese, & sour cream.	**Favor** goat's milk and ghee. **Reduce** all other dairy.
Fruits	**Favor** avocados, apricots bananas, cherries, and mangoes. **Reduce** apples, pomegranates and cranberries.	**Favor** exceptionally sweet fruits. **Reduce** grapefruit, sour berries and other sour fruits.	**Favor** apples and pears. **Reduce** bananas, avocados, coconuts and melons.
Vegetables	**Favor** asparagus, beets and carrots. **Reduce** sprouts and cabbage.	**Favor** asparagus, cucumbers, potatoes, broccoli & green beans. **Reduce** tomatoes, peppers, onions and radishes.	**Favor** all vegetables **except** tomatoes, potatoes and water chestnuts.
Beans	**Favor** mung beans, lentils & tofu occasionally. **Reduce** all others.	**Favor** all except lentils.	**Favor** all except black lentils, kidney beans and soybeans.
Grains	**Favor** rice, oats & wheat. **Reduce** barley, corn, millet, buckwheat and rye.	**Favor** rice, wheat, barley and oats. **Reduce** corn, millet, buckwheat, rye and yeasted bread.	**Favor** barley, corn, millet, buckwheat, and rice. **Reduce** wheat.
Sweeteners	**Favor** all sweeteners.	**Favor** all sweeteners except molasses.	**Favor** honey. **Reduce** all other sweeteners.
Oils	**Favor** all oils.	**Favor** olive, sunflower and coconut oils. **Reduce** sesame and corn oils.	**Favor** almond and sunflower oils in small quantities. **Reduce** all others.
Spices	**Favor** cardamom, cinnamon, cloves, cumin, garlic, ginger, mustard seed, black pepper and salt.	**Favor** coriander, turmeric and fennel. **Reduce** salt and hot spices like ginger, pepper and mustard seed.	**Favor** all spices. **Reduce** salt.

TWENTY ATTRIBUTES (GUNAS) AND THEIR ACTIONS

Attribute	Vata	Pitta	Kapha	Actions
Heavy	↓	↓	↑	Increases bulk nutrition and heaviness, creates dullness and lethargy.
Light	↑	↑	↓	Helps digestion, reduces bulk, cleanses, creates freshness and alertness.
Slow	↓	↓	↑	Creates sluggishness, slow action, relaxation & dullness.
Sharp	↑	↑	↓	Immediate effect, promotes sharpness, quick understanding, creates ulcers.
Cold	↑	↓	↑	Creates cold, numbness, contraction, unconsciousness, fear and insensitivity.
Hot	↓	↑	↓	Promotes heat, digestion, cleansing, expansion, inflammation and anger.
Oily	↓	↑	↑	Creates smoothness, moisture, lubrication, vigor, compassion and love.
Dry	↑	↓	↓	Increases dryness, absorption, constipation, nervousness and insomnia.
Slimy	↓	↑	↑	Decreases roughness, increases smoothness, love & care.
Rough	↑	↓	↓	Causes cracking of skin & bones. Creates carelessness and rigidity.
Dense	↓	↓	↑	Promotes solidity, density & strength.
Liquid	↓	↑	↑	Dissolves & liquifies, promotes salivation, compassion and cohesiveness.
Soft	↓	↑	↑	Creates softness, delicacy, relaxation, tenderness, love and care.
Hard	↑	↓	↑	Increases hardness, strength, rigidity.
Static	↓	↓	↑	Promotes stability, obstruction, support, constipation and faith.
Mobile	↑	↑	↓	Promotes motion, shakiness, restlessness and lack of faith.
Subtle	↑	↑	↓	Pierces, penetrates subtle capillaries, increases emotions and feelings.
Gross	↓	↓	↑	Causes obstruction and obesity.
Cloudy	↓	↓	↑	Heals fractures, causes lack of clarity and perception.
Clear	↑	↑	↓	Pacifies, creates isolation and diversion.

(↑ = increases, ↓ = decreases)

102

Nutrition for the Equestrian Athlete

As an athlete, you will benefit the most from creating a chemically and energetically balanced nutritional base as detailed in Ayurveda, and then further fine-tuning your eating habits to support your specific fitness regimens. You can best support your body before and after strenuous exercise by eating complex carbohydrates, because your body converts carbohydrates into energy more efficiently than fats or proteins. Carbohydrates are broken down into glucose during digestion, and then converted into energy and glycogen. The glycogen is stored in your muscles and liver for future use. During exercise, the stored glycogen is converted back into glucose to provide you with additional energy as you need it.

Complex carbohydrates provide you with a convenient source of prolonged, high-octane energy to fuel you through your workout and throughout your day.

▌ Carbohydrates will provide you with 40-50% of your energy requirement during the early stages of moderate exercise.

▌ Excess carbohydrates are stored as fat.

▌ Carbohydrates are found in potatoes, corn, and other vegetables, pasta, rice, beans, peas, breads, cereals and other grains.

▌ Many high-carbohydrate foods are also great sources of fiber.

Needed fats are converted into energy-providing glycerol and fatty acids. Unfortunately, excess fatty acids are easily stored as, you guessed it ... body fat, the nemesis of modern man and woman that lurks behind every morsel of food that tastes even remotely edible and the taskmaster that forces you to spend endless hours huffing and puffing and sweating into utter exhaustion....

There is a method to the madness of burning fat. Workouts can be highly effective fat-burning tools if you exercise wisely. The key is to exercise in a manner that increases your use of fat as fuel. Using fat as energy depends upon the intensity and duration of the exercise, and on your fitness level:

▌ You will burn more fat during moderate aerobic exercise than during strenuous exercise. Your body uses fat as its primary fuel during low and moderate intensity aerobic exercise. High intensity aerobic exercise causes your body to shift toward anaerobic metabolism and switch from consuming fat energy to carbohydrate energy as your primary fuel. Free fatty acid metabolism will fuel up to 50% of your energy requirement during moderate aerobic exercise such as fast-walking, jogging or cycling.

▌ Your body fat cells will begin to shrink in size after 20 minutes of moderate exercise, and you will use fat as a primary fuel after 1 hour of prolonged moderate aerobic exercise.

▌ The fit athlete will use fat for energy more rapidly and efficiently than the unfit athlete.

Protein is used in building muscle and lean tissue, and to some extent, provides energy. Contrary to popular belief, protein plays only a supportive role in muscle building. It is the combination of physical training and your body's use of total calories and quality nutrients that creates muscle. Exercise will not normally increase your need for protein, except in extreme cases such as those of bodybuilders or marathon runners.

▌ Extra protein is stored as body fat.

▌ Excess protein can deprive you of more efficient energy fuels, and can lead to dehydration as it increases the amount of

103

water required to eliminate your body's waste products.

▌ A diet of 10-12% protein is sufficient to meet all of your health and fitness needs, and can be met simply by eating a variety of foods.

▌ Protein is found in fish, meats, poultry, beans, peas, eggs, nuts, seeds, and soy products.

Eating a varied diet of nutrient and energy rich foods that are balancing to you will assure you of sufficient amounts of vitamins and minerals during normal daily activities. There is no evidence that eating extra vitamins will increase your performance level. However, minerals play a critical role in fitness and performance, and are affected by prolonged exercise. Strenuous exercise will deplete your body of sodium, potassium, iron and calcium. These minerals should be replenished by eating normally after exercise or an event.

Avoid excessive amounts of sodium, including salt tablets, and minimize (or eliminate) any use of electrolyte drinks. When you sweat, you naturally increase the salt concentration in your body and lower your water content. Excess sodium will absorb additional water from your body cells causing weak muscles, and will lower your potassium level, which is needed to regulate muscle activity.

Women athletes are often prone to iron deficiency, and may find it necessary to supplement iron in their diet. Iron serves to transport oxygen in your blood and muscles. Iron deficiency anemia impairs oxygen transport, which will decrease your aerobic performance and cause you to tire very easily. If you suspect you are iron deficient, contact your physician for testing.

Water is the most critical nutrient for any athlete. Water is present in all of your body's cells, tissues and organs. It transports your body's nutrients and waste products, lubri-

cates your tissues and digestive tract, lubricates and cushions your joints, and regulates your body temperature. That is an impressive job description.

Any equestrian-athlete can be prone to dehydration, which is the excessive loss of your body's fluids. Your body loses water primarily through sweating. You may be surprised to know that the next greatest amount of fluid loss is through breathing (water exhaled as vapor). To prevent dehydration and maximize your performance, you should start every exercise and event fully hydrated, and should replace lost body fluids by drinking water or diluted fruit juice at frequent intervals.

▌ A water loss of just 5% can reduce your performance capacity by 20-30%.

▌ The initial symptoms of dehydration are thirst, weakness, and then fatigue.

▌ Sodas, coffee and tea are not acceptable hydrating fluids. They contain caffeine and sugar, both of which contribute to dehydration. Caffeine acts as a diuretic, causing increased water excretion, and sugar requires additional water to properly absorb into your body's cells.

How do you know you are exercising moderately? An easy rule of thumb is if you cannot talk during exercise, you are working too intensely, so slow down. If you can sing, you are exercising too slowly, so speed up and work a little harder.

You have the facts, now let's use your nutrition knowledge to maximize your exercise performance:

▌ Your pre-workout meal should be high in complex carbohydrates and low in sugar and fat. Eating sugar before exercise or an event will not give you extra energy. It will hinder your performance by triggering a surge of insulin, which approximately 30 minutes later will cause a sharp drop in your blood sugar level and lead to fatigue.

▌ Drink plenty of water before, during and after your workout. Take frequent sips of water during exercise to keep yourself hydrated. If you wait until you are thirsty, then your performance level has already dropped.

▌ Eat a small carbohydrate-rich snack within 90 minutes after your workout to replace the fuel you burned during exercise and to aid in the recovery process necessary after every workout. A piece of fruit or a glass of juice and some whole grain crackers will suffice.

NUTRITIONAL STRATEGY FOR COMPETITIVE EQUESTRIAN EVENTS

The typical diet of today's rider-competitor at equine events is inadequate to meet the physical and mental demands of competition. The food offered at many concessions and fast food restaurants is usually high in fat, low in quality nutrients and fiber, and contributes only cheap calories incapable of sustaining an adequate energy level throughout the day.

During competition, various factors combine to drain your energy reserves more rapidly than normal and diminish your performance:

▌ Competitors endure elevated emotional stress levels throughout the day, with numerous high-stress peaks when involved in several events.

▌ Repeated physical and mental demands create an additional drain. Riding events require heightened mental awareness and focus, balance, muscular endurance, and occasionally strength and cardiovascular endurance.

▌ Events are often spread throughout the day, allowing you little time to leave the

grounds for a nutritious meal. The amount of time between breakfast and evening meals is longer. Both factors demand that your energy reserves last longer than usual.

▌ Both hot and cold weather can increase the loss of your body fluids.

Your nutritional goal during competition is to maintain a high and consistent energy level throughout the entire day. This will help you to remain mentally and physically sharp, and will give you a competitive edge in facing the myriad of challenges you will encounter. You can effectively manage your energy level by formulating a simple nutrition strategy:

▌ Begin by drinking plenty of water at least two days in advance. This will help ensure that you are fully hydrated when you begin you competition.

▌ The morning of your competition, drink plenty of water. Eat a breakfast of balancing foods that are high in carbohydrates, and low in fat and fiber. The reduced amount of fiber will speed up your digestion, and help you avoid an upset stomach during your events.

▌ During the day, drink plenty of water. Eat small, high-quality, high-carbohydrate snacks between your events or every two hours. You may drink some diluted fruit juice. Diluting the fruit juice will compensate for the juice's sugar content which requires your body to use additional water to absorb the sugar. Prepare or buy your snack foods ahead of time and keep them on hand in a cooler in a convenient location such as your trailer or stall.

105

3

The Mental Advantage

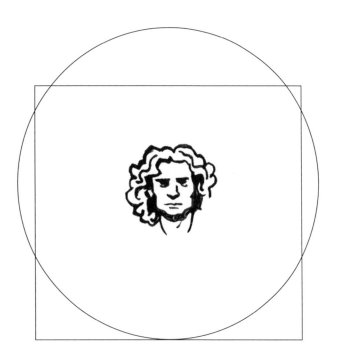

THE MENTAL ADVANTAGE

Equine Sports Psychology with Dr. Margot Nacey

THE ACTIVE PARTNERSHIP of human and horse relies extensively upon highly fragile and essential pathways of communication. These pathways carry all of the freely exchanged thoughts, sensations and emotions manifested in the form of cues and reactions that enable horse and rider to interact and perform. Only through free-flowing two-way communication can the horse-rider partnership learn, develop and reach a level of understanding necessary for success. Unfortunately, open communication can easily be disrupted and blocked, resulting in a performance breakdown.

The problem is that effective communication can only exist when horse and rider are interacting in a calm and harmonious state. This creates a difficult challenge when you consider that the larger-stronger member of this partnership is acutely tactile and sensitive, therefore easily affected by the slightest change in the rider's mental and physical conditions. Mental disruptions occur in the form of anxiety and, if left unchecked, can evolve into the more destructive conditions of fear and anger.

Anxiety can be defined as a state of feeling similar to fear, but without an identifiable cause. Anxiety can exist in a generalized state that affects your life on a daily basis over an extended period of time. It can also exist in a situational state and affect the performance of a specific task. When anxiety is situational it is described as "performance anxiety." Its effect on competitive performance depends upon the existing anxiety you bring to the situation and on the stress-causing demands of competition. Performance anxiety can affect you in number of subtle ways or it can quickly push you into an extreme debilitating state through a chain reaction of symptomatic growth.

It is possible to effectively control and overcome your anxieties by improving your mental self-awareness and by developing preventative-therapeutic mental techniques.

The Mental Advantage is a mental practice program developed by Margot Nacey, Ed.D., a licensed clinical psychologist, competitive rider and pioneer equestrian sports psychologist. This proven program is designed to help you conquer your performance anxiety, increase your self-awareness and improve your ability to focus under pressure. Through consistent mental practice you can be on top of your mental game.

BUILD A REDUCED-STRESS FOUNDATION

Performance anxiety is specific to a given situation, however it is easily intensified by unrelated stress sources present in other areas of your life. Existing stress and significant changes in your life combine to elevate your overall anxiety level and contribute to your performance anxiety level. Consequently, you must reduce the level of stress in your life outside of competitive sports and create a solid mental-emotional foundation before you can successfully take on your performance anxiety. Any significant event, whether good or bad, can cause additional stress in your life. Stress-causing events usually are changes that have taken place within the last year. Examples of significant life-changes include marriage, divorce, death of a friend or loved one, surgery, financial difficulties, change of job, relocation of residence, and difficulties in primary relationships.

The first step in building a reduced stress life is to identify the clues to your significant life-stressors:

▌ You eat too little or eat too much.

▌ You sleep too little or sleep too much.

▌ You're experiencing a loss of energy.

■ You're experiencing a lack of interest in things that normally interest you.

■ You're experiencing a lack of concentration.

■ You dwell on repetitive compulsive thoughts such as:

"I must not fail at anything. I won't do things unless I can do them well."

"I should have done that better."

"I can't do anything right."

"I can't ever please anyone."

"I wish I could change, but I can't."

"Everything must be in exactly the right order. Every detail must be perfect."

■ You "catastrophize" large and insignificant events into potential disasters.

The influence of change in your life can be overwhelmingly powerful. We tend to discount the power of life-changes because society supports the notion that feeling and emotions are secondary to and unrelated to our level of functioning. These feelings and emotions must be dealt with before they intensify your anxiety and evolve into negative visualization and into a destructive pattern of self-fulfilling prophecy.

While you cannot and do not want to avoid certain changes, you can learn to develop a healthy perspective and deal with change productively. Facing the problem is far healthier that denial or running away. When you are stressed and your emotional temperature is running high, the best strategy is to be kind to yourself:

■ Recognize your own limits of time and mental resources. Establish priorities and eliminate the low priority tasks. Use realistic scheduling.

■ Remind yourself of the positives in your life. Negative self-talk can turn into a self-fulfilling prophecy.

■ Slow down and allow yourself to relax. Tackle one task at a time.

■ Don't deny the existence of your problems. Recognize them and take constructive steps to deal with your problems by looking at them objectively, setting goals and developing a rational step-by-step problem-solving strategy.

■ Set realistic expectations. Expectations that are too high can lead to frustration and depression. It's healthy to strive for perfection as long as you accept the final reality that you can never achieve it.

■ Allow yourself to develop to your full potential as a competitor and as a person by choosing a healthier lifestyle. Consistent exercise, good nutrition and a positive mental practice will help you follow a more productive life direction.

■ Promote your rational thoughts such as:

"There's nothing to worry about."

"I'm going to be o.k."

"Take it one step at a time."

"I know I can complete these tasks."

"I know I can survive this."

"I've survived much worse than this."

"I'll give it my best effort and that is good enough."

Seek out and discover the logical, productive lesson from each situation. You can learn and benefit from any situation, good or bad.

IDENTIFY PERFORMANCE ANXIETY

There is no feeling quite like teaching your horse a new skill or riding in the show ring. For both horse and rider, competition serves as evidence of the commitment and effort put into achieving peak performance. You have prepared your horse and yourself thoroughly, with each step of your training and practice aimed toward making your next performance a success.

However, some aspects of competition are difficult to anticipate and prepare for. Every rider has experienced "butterflies" in their stomach prior to entering the arena, or had a great ride in the warm-up arena only to have their performance fall apart when it counted. How do you prepare to be not only physically ready for competition, but mentally prepared as well?

Peak mental performance begins with identifying the signs of performance anxiety. The majority of performance anxiety symptoms are initially very subtle and gradually become more apparent as your anxiety builds. Unless you are adept at identifying your initial stress symptoms you can remain unaware of your rising stress level until it reaches an advanced state. When your anxiety grows to this point, it is more difficult to control and can have an extreme debilitating effect on your performance.

Learning to recognize the initial clues to your performance anxiety will enable you to identify mounting tension in the early stages and take positive action to alleviate it before it gets out of hand. Initial anxiety symptoms can begin up to 10 days prior to competition. Initial clues to performance anxiety are:

▌ Sleep disturbances such as a difficulty falling asleep, waking abruptly or an inability to fall back asleep. You may find yourself sleeping too little or too much.

▌ Bad dreams such as dreams of conflict and nightmares.

▌ Vague feelings of distress. You experience mood swings, feel anxious and a loss of control. You are uncomfortable with yourself and are hypersensitive to criticism.

▌ You obsess on negative events such as the last time you fell off of your horse, blew a lead, forgot your course pattern, etc. You

agonize over past poor performances and project future poor performances. This can create negative self-fulfilling prophecies.

The next step is to develop an awareness of your body's physical tension signals. These are warnings that your body is internalizing mental stress and worry. In most individuals, these physical tension signals will occur repeatedly in the same body location over a period of time. This area of your body is known as your "tension zone" and serves as a reliable and timely clue to building internalized anxiety. A stiff neck or a sore back may be a significant clue that you have internalized your pre-competition performance anxiety. Your body's physical tension signals include:

▌ Aches and pains.

▌ Numbness in your hands and feet.

▌ Somatic symptoms such as headaches, stomach and gastrointestinal pains, and skin, respiratory and cardiovascular disorders.

Performance anxiety symptoms may occur during your warm-up or as you enter the ring. Symptoms commonly include muscle tension, sweating, dry mouth, irritability, loss of focus, excessive worry, loss of short-term memory, dizziness, difficulty in breathing and heart palpitations. The dreaded scenario may unfold like this:

It is 4 to 5 hours before your event. You have plenty of time, yet you are feeling irritable and you snap at a friend for an insignificant mistake. You become a little disoriented and your memory is fuzzy. Now, what were you going to do next? And where in the #?#!! did you leave that !#@#! hoof pick? You're feeling dizzy, so you sit down for a moment. You fail to notice that your breathing is becoming shallower.

It is one hour before your event. You begin warming up your horse. You're worrying that the competition is tough, the arena is a little soggy, and your horse is not performing the way you want. Tension is building in your muscles resulting in a lack of flexibility throughout your body. Of course, your horse immediately senses your stiffness and tense nerves and reacts negatively by tensing up himself. You soon notice that your horse is not warming up properly and you become more tense, and again your horse senses this and responds with increased tension, which you notice … and so on.

It is 15 minutes before your event. You first notice that your stomach is starting to feel queasy, but soon your lunch is doing things never intended for the human body. You make a mad dash for the nearest bathroom. You're becoming more tense and stiff, your mouth is now completely dry, and you're sweating as if you were doing the tango in a sauna. Unfortunately, there's more. You've developed a splitting headache, and it has become impossible for you to concentrate … and this is no time for a loss of focus. Your breathing is increasingly short and shallow, your heart is beating rapidly (heart palpitations), and the only thing you're able to visualize is you and your horse doing the worst "crash-and-burn" this horse show has ever seen!

It is the end of your event and you are leaving the arena. Your ride went poorly. You feel a loss of energy and you are unable to focus on the good parts of your ride. You are thinking only of all the things you and your horse did wrong.

Many equestrians experience some or all of the above stress symptoms, engage in negative visualization, and in an example of self-fulfilling prophecy, set the stage for yet another frustrating performance. However, this does not have to be you. It is possible to climb out of negative self-fulfilling prophecies

and create better performance and a healthier life by listening to your body, particularly your tension zones, identifying mounting tension in its initial stages and taking positive action to conquer your anxiety.

Many trainers and coaches agree that riders only achieve 60–70% of their true ability in the show ring. The other 30–40% is lost to stage fright or to real physical fear. At all levels of equestrian competition, the equestrian athletes who are able to master their anxiety and focus on the present moment are the ones who will achieve success in their performance and will have the Mental Advantage over their competitors.

CONQUER PERFORMANCE ANXIETY

Until recently we referred to our brain's two different hemispheres as our left and right sides of the brain. Dr. Milton Erickson referred to the left side as the conscientious mind and the right side he called the unconscientious mind. Today, we look at this as two ways of processing information. The left side of our brain, or our conscientious mind, is our logic, linear thoughts, sequencing, and our ability to analyze. It is a major information processing system. It is what allows us to balance our checkbooks. Our educational systems typically reinforce this type of mental processing. The right side of our brain, or our unconscientious mind is our intuition and sense of humor. It is spontaneous and sees the full picture. It is the home of our imagination and creativity.

Let's say you are observing a horse performing in the arena. Your "left brain" sees the details and gives a literal account of the horse's performance: The horse stopped here, went 4 strides to the left, jumped the vertical, then to the oxer, etc. Your "right brain" sees the horse being groomed, warmed up and then being ridden in the arena, notes the horse's mood, and sees the horse being cooled out and returned to the barn. Both ways of processing are important to us, but until recently we were unaware of how to communicate with the right brain method of communication.

Elite athletes often speak of being in "The Zone." The Zone is a state of mind where a sense of feel, rhythm and balance are at an optimum with seemingly little effort. This is perhaps a state largely created by the broader processing of the unconscientious mind, or the right brain.

The right hemisphere of your brain is sometimes called the "natural brain", the one you were born with. Dr. Erickson discovered ways to effectively communicate with the natural brain. Your natural brain cannot be commanded or forced, it must be spoken to gently through metaphor, suggestion, use of an image or by thinking in pictures. It is through these forms of communication that certain techniques have been proven to be effective in giving an athlete's body the messages needed to calmly implement the detailed skills taught in the athlete's left brain.

It is from this perspective that Dr. Nacey has seen so much success in assisting competitive riders to overcome performance anxiety and fear to achieve new levels of success in their performance. The following techniques are used by Dr. Nacey to assist clients to achieve success in life and in the show ring.

Self-Hypnosis

The word "hypnosis" usually conjures up images of magic acts where people are hypnotized and ordered to do embarrassing things like strut like a chicken and bark like a dog, things they would never contemplate if they were in control. The true technique of hypnosis is quite different from this entertaining misconception. Self-hypnosis is used to impart a deeper sense of control and self-reliance in your thought processes at the very times that you feel the least in control. This

technique will help you to distract yourself from anxiety and to focus on the present job at hand in a stressful situation such as the show ring.

The object of self-hypnosis is three-fold:

1. Instill feelings of well-being, safety and confidence, and to promote concentration and focus. In the sport of equestrian competition it is important that you, the rider, feel relaxed, centered and confident. This sense of confidence is instantaneously communicated to your horse, forming a crucial part of your dynamic, for it enables belief in each other's decisions and makes harmonious movements possible. Installation of a process for maintaining feelings of well-being and safety will allow you to limit negative thought patterns and to stay focused in the present moment during a competitive performance.

2. Allow freedom from overwhelming performance anxiety and distraction, and freedom to reach the goals you have set for yourself.

3. Build your self-confidence.

Whether riding for pleasure on the trail or working to improve competitive performance, self-hypnosis and the other recommended techniques can enhance your ability to concentrate and perform effectively with your horse. When riders use this method of self-hypnosis, most are able to reach the point where they feel calm, focused and able to smoothly execute the riding tasks they are asked to do. Athletes refer to this state as "being in the flow," or at the point where they feel calm, safe, aware, and in control, both in and out of competition. You can enjoy the entire training and competitive experience. As your focus is enhanced, you will become less dependent on other's judgments and able to ignore ringside chatter and distractions. Your increased enjoyment will enable you to let go of the "need" to win and will free you to have fun, grow and allow your body to respond to the best of its ability in a relaxed manner.

The experience of self-hypnosis is unique for each person. It is designed to give an individual method of mental protection and control in particularly stressful situations. Since that control belongs to you when you're utilizing the technique, your use of self-hypnosis will be unique to you, suited to your own particular needs. Once you have mastered the technique, it can be used anywhere, anytime and in a variety of situations. For maximum benefit, contact a licensed mental health professional to assist you in the initial training of this self-hypnosis technique.

To prepare for the technique, choose a comfortable chair in a quiet location. Now, let's begin:

■ Place both feet on the floor. Take deep, slow breaths, allowing yourself to relax and let go of things that might be on your mind. Consider a color that calms you. You can do this with your eyes open or closed.

■ Now that you feel comfortable and relaxed, picture in your mind a place where you feel safe and calm. This is your "safe place". It can be a real place you have visited, a place from a dream, or a place you read about or saw in a movie. Please choose a safe place that does not involve horses. Although a horse related place may feel safe now, it may trigger anxious feelings when you are in a stressful situation around horses or are preparing to perform in the arena. Examples of safe spots are your warm bed, a tree house with the ladder pulled up, a cozy chair by the fire on a cold evening, or a hammock swinging in the summer breeze.

■ Now that you have chosen your safe place, enjoy the process of going there. Take your time; if it doesn't come now, it may come later today or tomorrow. Once you are there, take a few moments to look around and note the sounds, smells and feel of the place. Note the time of day. Open all of your senses to record in your mind the flavor of your safe spot:

■ What do you see? Is there grass or trees? What colors do you see?

■ What do you smell? Is there freshly cut grass? Are flowers blooming?

■ What sounds do you hear – the wind through the trees, birds chirping, or children laughing?

■ What does your safe place feel like? Can you feel a breeze on your face, or perhaps the feel of warm sand between your toes?

■ Take some time to enjoy your safe space and allow yourself to feel very calm, very secure and very peaceful.

■ Now look around. Is there anything in your safe place that you can bring back with you… something that would symbolize your safety and immediately remind you of your safe place? It can be anything you choose from your safe place: a flower, a leaf, your dog's whisker, the smell of spaghetti, anything. When you have chosen that one thing, picture it carefully in your mind. The item you have chosen to represent your safe place is called an "artifact". It may take 1 to 5 sessions to formally install your safe place and its artifact. Spend a few more moments in your safe place and simply enjoy it. Take your time. Remember, you have all the time you need. When you are ready, slowly and gently open your eyes and return to where you are.

In order to be able to rely on your new technique, you should practice "going to" your safe place in your mind approximately five times a day. This can be done anywhere and anytime: over cereal in the morning or sitting at your desk. One of the best times to practice is when you are putting your head down on your pillow. A time between wake and sleep, it will be very easy to "go to" your safe place.

Gradually, your use of this technique will allow you to utilize this tool whenever you need to relax and refresh yourself. The more you practice your self-hypnosis, the more you train your unconscious mind to be your friend and allow your body to respond in an appropriate and trained fashion. This technique will enable a rider's well trained body to act in the way it has been taught to do: naturally, spontaneously and in good balance. When your feelings of anxiety and intimidation are replaced with a sense of confidence, you will be able to ride your horse in a natural manner with an increased awareness of your horse's movement and rhythm. With this sense of calm and confidence transmitting to your horse, the free-flowing two-way communication between horse and rider can be enhanced, allowing each of you to perform to your best potential and to give your best effort.

EMDR Therapy

EMDR, or Eye Movement Desensitization and Reprocessing, was developed by Dr. Francine Shapiro in 1989. Since then, thousands of mental health professionals have been trained in this technique. The use of EMDR can benefit a rider who has been injured and mentally or physically traumatized. Physical trauma can cause deep-seated fear, panic attacks, flashbacks, depression and loss of self-esteem. Everyone experiences fear differently; what may cause one rider fear may not cause another rider fear. EMDR therapy can work to change the fearful memory and install positive, confident responses to the same situation by changing the rider's perception of body memories, the trigger situation, level of fear and degree of depression.

Dr. Shapiro discovered that when the eyes moved from one side of the head to the other, in a bi-lateral fashion, there was a physiologi-

cal change. Dr. Shapiro was planting bulbs in her garden when she noted that as she moved her eyes left to right and right to left and then the other way again, she could not remember her immediate prior thought. This was the beginning of EMDR.

Researchers have learned that people who have had psychological trauma often have body memories of that event. These memories seem to be resistant to change and are often triggered by situations similar to the one that created the trauma. Neuropsychologists discovered through SPECT brain imaging that traumatic memories seem to be located on the right side of the brain. After EMDR treatment, these images are not in the same location. Further studies suggest that eye movements may help traumatic memories move from the right side of the brain to the left side of the brain, which serves as a storage area for conscious information and enables you to consciously process these memories. You take the psychological or emotional memory and make it an objective memory. You know the trauma occurred, but it does not hold the power it once did. You thereby transform the trauma, reduce the associated physical symptoms, dissipate the flashbacks and produce positive long-lasting change.

EMDR is especially useful with equestrians because of the nature of the sport and its inherent physical danger. Over the last 20 years, Dr. Nacey's most common type of sports psychology clients have been riders who have sustained physical injury from some type of horse-related accident. EMDR is particularly helpful to riders because of the impact of body memories. When you are traumatized, your adrenalin is swiftly activated and imprints the event in your memory system. This imprinted memory can sometimes stay frozen in time only to be continually relived or triggered by witnessing a similar event. Body memories can reappear in the heat of competition or in other times of stress. These memories can be accompanied with a feeling of uneasiness or in some cases full-blown panic. With the help of EMDR treatment, many riders with serious injury have successfully returned to competition with renewed confidence and feelings of safety. They feel less tension in their bodies and are free from the anxiety that inhibited their performance.

EMDR has other uses for the equestrian. Riders often remember more of their disappointing rides and have difficulty remembering their good rides. EMDR therapy can be used to reinforce positive memories and positive future direction, and it can also be used to establish a safe place for self-hypnosis. If you are interested in EMDR, contact a mental health professional who is certified in EMDR therapy.

Imagery and Your Calming Color

Many people can enhance their sense of security and relaxation through the use of imagery. Imagery consists of focusing on your senses of smell, taste, hearing and touch while visualizing a pleasant scene, and then utilizing the calming effects. A highly effective imagery exercise is to envision your calming color or calming image. Like colors, images can help your body to relax and focus. The more detailed the image, the more effect it has on you. You can imagine running your fingers over a smooth rock or smelling the raspberry pie your grandmother baked. One of Dr. Nacey's clients rubs a smooth image rock, which she found in a stream, to put herself in the mood to rest and sleep. She hears water flowing over the rock, making it smoother and smoother.

Another client of Dr. Nacey's focuses on her calming color as she works with young horses, both on the ground and in the saddle. She pairs a quiet voice with the image of her calming color and the horses relax immediately. If, during the course of training, the horses become upset, she returns to her calming color image.

The following exercise can be performed before your riding lesson, your pre-competition warm-up, your performance, or whenever you feel tense and insecure.

Mental Advantage Exercise

1. Go to your safe place. It is your private sanctuary; you can use it to help you focus on your calming image or calming color. Choose a color that creates a feeling of warmth, calmness and security within you. Imagine breathing in that calming color, and as it fills every pore of your body with a smoothing peaceful feeling, imagine putting all distracting thoughts in a hole in the ground or in the dumpster.

2. Take a sheet of paper and draw a square 2 inches across. Color your calming color inside the square. As you color, try to experience the feelings your color brings to your senses. Some people smell their calming color while others hear it. It is up to you as to how you use your calming color or image.

3. Look into your color. Go, squint your eyes and focus at it. Maybe it has hue or texture. Close your eyes and try to imagine your color. Try some deep breathing as you imagine your color. Breathe in your calming color. Breathe out tension.

4. Your color calms and soothes you. It makes you feel safe and warm. Try to imagine your calming color surrounding you and protecting you from all harm and negative energy.

5. Each night as you lie in bed, envision and feel your calming color and its soothing effects.

Once you are able to imagine your calming color quickly and consistently, perform this exercise every time you ride your horse. You may notice that your thoughts of your calming color, calming image, artifact or safe place also relax your horse.

Positive Visualization

Visualization can be defined as the innate

ability to imagine yourself successfully or unsuccessfully completing an act. When used correctly, positive visualization can serve as mental support in the process of rapid problem solving. Visualization is not a new phenomenon. Native Americans have used visualization for hundreds of years as an important part of their cultures.

Modern precedents exist as well. In 1972, an Australian psychologist, Alan Richardson, completed a study in visualization now recognized as a classic in sports psychology. Richardson divided a number of basketball players into 3 groups. For 20 days, one group practiced making free throws, one group visualized making free throws, and the results were surprising. The group of players who visualized making baskets easily compiled the best free throw shooting percentage and the highest score.

This study has since been replicated many times by other psychologists with the same results: Visualization enhances skill. This does not suggest that visualization can replace the fundamentals of training. Visualization does not replace the experience itself. All of these basketball players had advanced basketball skills before they participated in the experiment. Mastery of the basic techniques and skills of your sport are necessary before visualization can be used effectively. Your best results will be attained by supplementing your training in the saddle with The Mental Advantage program, including positive visualization.

The practiced use of deep breathing, relaxation and stress reduction will build a positive foundation by placing you in a receptive state of awareness and inner balance conducive to productive imagery. You must be in a relaxed state and be able to focus in a relaxed manner for visualization to be successful. No lasting benefits can be derived from any mental practice program until you are able to induce a true state of deep relax-

ation. To do this, you must practice a little each day.

To begin visualizing, close your eyes and simply see what is behind your eyelids. Try this for 4–5 minutes at a time for a couple of days. Gradually, you will see more color and images.

Not everyone is successful with visualization and not everyone visualizes the same way. Some people "feel" visualization while others are auditory visualizers ... they actually hear the rhythm of their horse's hoof beats instead of seeing it. One way to see what kind of visualizer you are is to try to remember your bedroom as a child. Close your eyes and see what comes up. Maybe you remember the color of the bedspread, maybe you smell the scent of fresh sheets, or maybe you hear the blinds blowing in the breeze. Practice on this familiar place and gradually you will come to know if you visualize at all and what type of visualizer you are. About 65% of people visualize, the rest may hear, smell, taste or feel. But almost everyone can visualize if they close their eyes and practice visualizing their bedroom immediately after doing the eyelids technique. You may be surprised what you learn about yourself.

Here are a few tips for effective positive visualization:

▍ Visualize yourself being in complete control of your performance. Break down your performance into smaller, individual steps and visualize each one.

▍ Write down affirmations of the skills you want to improve on, such as "keep my heels down, stay balanced and centered in the saddle, or keep my eyes up and looking forward". This forms a written agreement with yourself that you can accomplish your specific goals. Symbolic visualization can assist you in your performance. If you are trying to prevent your chest from collapsing and your shoulders from rolling forward during the canter depart, then imagine your chest being pulled skyward by a string from the clouds and your shoulders being gently pushed back by a summer breeze.

■ Use all of your senses when visualizing. Attempt to see, hear, touch, taste and smell your images.

■ Visualize in color instead of black and white. The more realistic your visualization, the better.

■ Always end your visualization on a positive note. If you make an error, correct it before you conclude.

■ Establish a regular visualization routine. Only through consistent practice will you become proficient at these techniques.

■ You have worked on the details at home. You are prepared. Don't worry about every excruciating detail during your performance. Be confident and allow your visualization and non-traditional thought processes to work for you.

Regular practice of these methods along with your safe place and artifact will help you to effectively use them any time you need to focus. When negative thoughts pop up, try these quick methods to dissuade them:

■ **Eye Roll.** This technique was first discovered in 1989 by Dr. Francis Shapiro. The eye roll, which is useful for about 60% of the population, can help you forget your immediate prior thought. Roll your eyes to the left, then up, then to the right, then down. That's it.

■ **Tapping.** If the negative thought persists, return to your safe place, focus on your artifact, and use a tapping sequence to interrupt your disturbing thoughts and help you to refocus in a more useful direction.

■ **Slowing Down.** Equestrian athletes often

complain that it is all going too fast. One way to help yourself balance and slow down is to focus on your artifact and then imagine a time when you were waiting – for a favorite restaurant to open, in line for concert tickets, or reflect on syrup being slowly poured over pancakes.

■ **Gaining Energy.** Sometimes you want to increase your rhythm and keep your horse lively and energized. When you do, try this: Focus on your artifact and then think of a time when you deliberately hurried to call a friend or to keep up with your dog on the leash as he rushes along the sidewalk, etc. You can also visualize a color that gives you a boost such as red or yellow.

Try this positive visualization exercise:

Mental Advantage Exercise

1. Choose any photo of you and your horse that you are proud of. It can be an action shot or a posed shot.

2. Find a quiet and calm place to practice.

3. Try going to your safe place. Focus on your artifact, calming color or image, and take a couple of slow deep breaths to place yourself in a receptive state of mind.

4. Look at your photo with a "soft eye", that is, keep your eyes slightly unfocused. Squinting slightly can help you maintain a "soft eye". Keep your artifact in your focus.

5. Close your eyes and imagine the photo in color and in as much detail as you can.

6. Acknowledge the good and successful qualities of you and your horse:

7. "My horse is very athletic and moves smoothly and gracefully."

8. "My horse has a beautiful neck and great conformation."

9. "We have a very balanced and collected canter."

10. "I ride with good balance in the saddle."

11. Acknowledge you and your horse's triumphs.

Allow yourself to be proud of your accomplishments.

For your visualization and imagery practice, you should have someone videotape your training sessions and your competitive performances so you can observe your riding in private. Most horse shows have a professional video service taping the competition or you can enlist a friend. Initially, you may be uncomfortable watching yourself on a video and will be overly self-critical. It often takes several viewings before you can relax and enjoy the viewing. One way to help yourself overcome self-criticism is to pretend you are blowing your errors out of your mind and body into a shiny red balloon. Blow hard and feel the tightness of the balloon with your fingertips. After you have put all of your self-criticism into the balloon, tie a knot at the bottom of the balloon. Focus on your breathing and feel the air come in and go out of your lungs. As your breath goes out, imagine letting go of the red balloon and watching it float far away out of your sight and out of your thoughts.

Once you can avoid extreme self-criticism, you are ready to begin using the video for productive visualization and imagery practice.

Mental Advantage Exercise

1. Sit down in a comfortable position in front of your VCR and television. Relax using deep breathing and the imagery techniques you have learned. Begin with your safe place, and then imagine your calming color.

2. Begin viewing your video. Play your video in slow motion, if possible. This will give you better control over the imagery and visualization process.

3. View with a "soft eye," that is, keep your eyes slightly unfocused as you watch your video. Squinting slightly can help you maintain a "soft eye."

4. Breathe slowly and rhythmically. If you get a negative thought or image, use the eye roll or tapping technique to dispose of it.

5. Concentrate on the positive aspects of your ride. Reward and affirm yourself aloud on the good points of your ride.

6. Occasionally pause your VCR and visualize what you just saw. If that portion of your ride includes an error on your part, then close your eyes and visualize the correction. If you become distracted, use your eye roll, artifact, tapping or imagery techniques to help yourself become focused again. You can also place more self-criticism in your red balloon and send it away again.

7. Always end a visualization exercise on a positive performance and positive thoughts, never on a negative performance or with self-critical negative thought.

It may take up to 7 or 8 visualization practice sessions before you become comfortable and proficient at the visualization-imagery process. The use of video will build your visualization skills and provide productive and feedback that will aid your use of positive imagery during competition. If you do not have a good ride on video, then get a copy of a successful professional ride and imagine yourself as the rider flowing in unison with the horse.

If you consistently practice your Mental Advantage program, you will be able to better prepare for competition by visualizing a successful ride and being calm, confident and aware. Visualize yourself successfully meeting your specific riding and competitive goals: staying balanced and centered in the saddle, maintaining good posture, cueing with precision, remembering your course pattern, and so on. Envision yourself competing in a calm but assertive manner, and smoothly handling any problem you encounter.

Goal Setting

Goals are a crucial part of your program to improve your skills and performance. However, when individuals choose idealistic goals and do not attain them, they typically feel badly, and then chastise themselves for failing and for not working hard enough. This quickly evolves into a negative cycle, which results in self-defeating behavior and increases performance anxiety. An obvious example of an idealistic goal is, "I want to win every horse show". This goal seems extreme, yet some competitors feel defeated and a failure unless they take 1st place.

To be a healthy competitor you must accept that you cannot control everything. You have no control over show conditions, subjective opinions, bad weather, spooky occurrences, your horse's soundness and countless other factors. It is not good enough to be good; you have to be flexible as well … when the wind blows, the bamboo bends.

Establishing realistic goals will help you develop a healthy and sustainable perspective towards competition. These goals will form the foundation of your mental practice program. Choose specific goals that you can control and realistically attain. For example, divide your goal to succeed at horse shows into more specific goals such as:

- Be relaxed prior to and during your performance.

- Maintain correct riding posture, especially lengthening your legs, lowering your heels and keeping your eyes forward, etc.

- Be precise in your seat and leg cues.

- Keep your horse moving straight and forward.

Dr. Nacey encourages all of her sports psychology clients to define their goals. Over the years she has discovered that the majority of riders set their goals too high. Goals should be realistic, flexible and set with your trainer. Form three to five sets of goals: one for you, one for your horse, one for you and your horse, one for work, one for family and relationships, and perhaps one for education. The trick is to correlate your goals so that one

set does not overlap another set. Be specific and passionate about your goals.

Once you have set your goals, daydream a little about them. Imagine how it would be a year from now. Imagine what you would be doing, feeling and wearing. Use your riding log to write down what it would be like a year from now for you and your horse.

Here are some tips in setting realistic goals:

- Choose specific and attainable short-term, mid-term and long-term goals. Write them down.

- State your goals only in positive terms such as, "I will be calm" or "I will remember my pattern", instead of in negative terms such as, "I won't panic" or "I won't blow my pattern".

- Visualize yourself successfully completing each step toward your goal.

- Consider time management. Have you allotted enough time to accomplish your goals?

- Gain useful insight into your goal development by asking for your trainer's input. The best time to discuss your goals with your trainer is when he/she can listen, not at the show, but long before. Be clear, honest and specific, and your trainer will do the same.

- Observe your peers at a similar level of preparation and expertise. Ask them how they reached that level of success.

- Keep a brief daily riding log. This will assist you in creating a more complete view of your goals and will help keep you focused on the facts and specific tasks.

THE MENTAL ADVANTAGE DURING COMPETITION

Here are some helpful tips for staying calm and focused during competition:

■ Maintain a consistent energy level by eating a high carbohydrate, low sugar, low fat diet and drinking plenty of water at least two days prior to and during the days you are competing.

■ If necessary, tell critical family members to stay home or away from the show during the days you are competing.

■ Stretch thoroughly before you mount your horse.

■ Use someone as a support system. This person should be a non-demanding friend whose knowledge and judgments you trust, such as your trainer.

■ Take your time warming up your horse. Use your relaxation techniques before your event. Don't wait until you feel tense. Listen for your tension signals; some people are unaware of the degree of tension in their body or in their behavior.

■ Visualize your ride before you enter the ring. Do not concentrate on the details; instead, focus on the essence of a smooth ride.

■ When the competitor before you encounters a problem (falls to the ground, misses the correct lead, knocks a pole or rail down, etc.), do not become distracted. Use your eye roll, tapping or artifact to remain completely focused on yourself, your horse and your game plan.

■ Ignore other competitors' negative emotions or comments, just as you ignore your left brain chatter. Use your relaxation techniques to construct a protective barrier around yourself and your horse. Do your eye roll, go to your safe place or focus on your artifact. There is usually a lot of useless chatter around the gate … ignore it.

■ Your self-esteem is never dependent on winning. You are a good rider whether you win or not.

■ Reward yourself and your horse on your improvements. Stick to your specific short-term goals and keep sight of your long-term goals.

■ Patience is invaluable. You can train yourself to develop patience. Gary Player, the famous golf pro, taught himself patience by finding the slowest drivers on the highway and staying behind them. When you teach yourself patience, you naturally teach the same to your horse. Now that is a worthy goal.

■ There will always be another horse show. Countless variable conditions exists that you cannot control, but you can choose to try again.

What if you experience an anxiety attack during your ride? How do you quickly salvage your ride and continue with your performance? If you have consistently practiced you mental program techniques, then you are capable of implementing an emergency strategy for regaining control of your performance:

■ Use your eye roll, tapping, calming color imagery or safe place artifact to regain control of your runaway negative thoughts.

■ Then focus on the mechanics of your ride. Break down the remaining portion of your performance into simple individual steps such as maintaining good balance, concentrating on your horse's stride and pace and maintaining a good rhythm, executing your commands smoothly, maintaining good posture, and so on.

To achieve full benefit you should practice all of the techniques in The Mental Advantage program twice a day for three or four weeks. Only through consistent practice and patience will you be able to use these natural calming and focusing methods when

121

you need them the most. Mastery of the techniques in The Mental Advantage will enable you to seize control of your mental and physical processes, and empower you to perform with more confidence.

You will utilize your energy more productively and efficiently, and you will develop an improved awareness of yourself and your surroundings. You will learn to live more comfortably in the present. Reality exists only in the here and now, not in the past, nor in the future. When competing, you must exist in the present, so that you can concentrate fully on your horse, yourself and your performance.

Consider the following possibility: Your months of physical preparation and mental practice are working for you. Your horse is trained and prepared, and you are focused and relaxed. You can now instantly call upon proven calming strategies if you need them. You are capable of harnessing the power of positive visualization and self-hypnosis to enhance your performance. You are now ready to be tested and you welcome the competitive experience because you have fun and always learn and improve from your performance. You feel empowered and you have the resources to handle any situation that may arise.

An anxious mind cannot exist

within a relaxed body.

EDMUND JACOBSEN
the father of
progressive relaxation

4 Appendix - Props

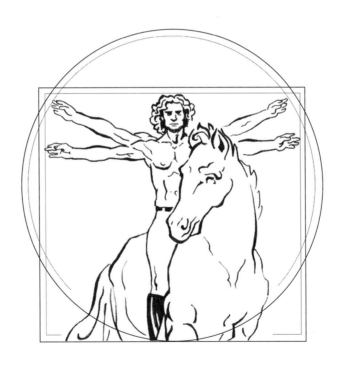

PROPS

BUILDING A BALANCE BOARD

A balance board is easy to construct. The supplies needed are:

1. 1 - 1" x 12" x 16" board
2. 1 - 2" x 2" x 15" board
3. 2 - 1/4" x 2" wood screws
4. wood glue
5. pencil
6. ruler or tape measure
7. hammer
8. screwdriver

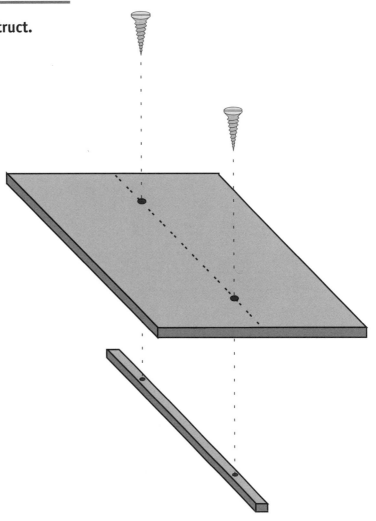

▌ Draw a line lengthwise down the middle of the board.

▌ Center two wood screws on the line and drive them through until they appear on the other side.

▌ Draw a line lengthwise down the middle of the 2" x 2", apply a bead of glue.

▌ Center the 2" x 2" on the 12" x 16" board and fasten tightly with the wood screws.

▌ Let it dry overnight before using.

THE PHYSIO-BALL

The physio-ball has become a valued component in a wide range of fitness workouts. Other common names for the physio-ball are the Theraball or Swiss-ball. It can be purchased at many major department stores and sporting goods stores.

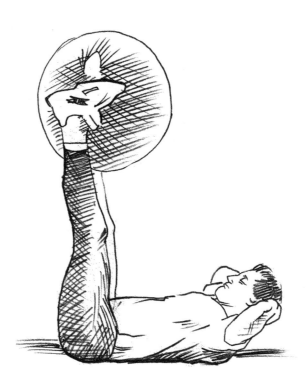

THE THERABAND

A simple exercise device constructed of rubber tubing, the theraband can be found in sporting goods stores and some department stores. If needed, contact your fitness professional for assistance in locating a theraband.

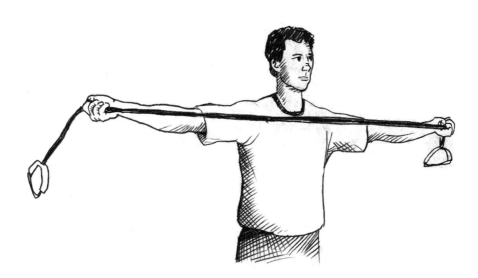

SOURCES

Anderson, Jennifer and Diane Preves.
Nutrition for the Athlete. Fort Collins,
CO: Colorado State University
Cooperative Extension, No. 9.362.

Cousens, Gabriel. **Conscious Eating**.
Patagonia, AZ: Essene Vision Books,
1997.

Svoboda, Robert E. **Prakriti: Your
Ayurvedic Constitution**. Bellingham,
WA: Sadhana Publications, 1998.

FITNESS NOTES